Beyond Slash, Burn,
and Poison

Beyond Slash, Burn, and Poison

TRANSFORMING BREAST CANCER STORIES INTO ACTION

MARCY JANE KNOPF-NEWMAN

RUTGERS UNIVERSITY PRESS
New Brunswick, New Jersey, and London

LIBRARY OF CONGRESS CATALOGING-IN-PUBLICATION DATA

Knopf-Newman, Marcy Jane.
  Beyond slash, burn, and poison : transforming breast cancer stories into
action / Marcy Jane Knopf-Newman.
     p.   cm.
  Includes bibliographical references and index.
  ISBN 0–8135–3470–4 (hardcover : alk. paper) — ISBN 0–8135–3471–2
(pbk : alk. paper)
    1. Breast—Cancer—Social aspects—United States. 2. Cancer patients'
writings, American. I. Title.
  RC280.B8K58 2004
  362.196′99449′0092273—dc22 2004000298

British Cataloging-in-Publication information for this book is available
from the British Library.

Copyright © 2004 by Marcy Jane Knopf-Newman

Excerpts from letters between Rachel Carson and Dorothy Freeman are from
Always, Rachel: The Letters of Rachel Carson and Dorothy Freeman, 1952–1964,
copyright © 1995 by Roger Allen Christie.

Excerpts from letters to and from Dr. George Crile are from *A Darker Ribbon:
Breast Cancer, Women, and Their Doctors in the Twentieth Century,* copyright © 1999
by Ellen Leopold.

Excerpt from letter to Paul Brooks was first published in *The House of Life: Rachel
Carson at Work,* copyright © 1972 by Paul Brooks.

All other letters from Rachel Carson are from *Rachel Carson: Witness for Nature,*
copyright © 1997 by Linda Lear.

Reprinted by permission of Frances Collin, Trustee u-w-o Rachel Carson.

Manufactured in the United States of America

This book is dedicated to the memory of my mother, Jane Gibbons-Knopf, whose struggle with breast cancer taught me about survival, and to my grandmother Marian Newman Gibbons, who taught me about the power of narratives.

I also dedicate this book to Karen Khale, whose presence reminds me why this work continues to be vital.

Contents

PREFACE

OFTEN WHEN I describe this book to people, they ask me, Why breast cancer? Why did I choose to focus on one particular type of cancer when the treatment and experience of all forms of the disease are remarkably similar? I chose to write about breast cancer for many intellectual and philosophical reasons; however, a personal experience frames the subject of *Beyond Slash, Burn, and Poison* for me.

The weekend I moved into my first-year college dormitory in the fall of 1987, my mother found two lumps in her left breast while performing a self-exam. It was a Friday night and my father and sister were with me—two thousand miles away. By Wednesday her doctors informed her that she had malignant cells, but neither physician uttered the words *breast cancer*. That turn of phrase comforted her at the time as she felt that "I can deal with a cell . . . but breast cancer is too big for me to deal with right now."[1] My mom thought about the kind of surgery she wanted to have for two weeks. Researching the latest findings in the library of UCLA, discussing her concerns with physicians, she had a difficult time weighing all the choices that lay before her. Initially she decided to have a lumpectomy followed by radiation. However, a physician friend recommended a modified radical mastectomy because of the tumor size; and on October 6, 1987, my mom had her left breast removed.

On what she called decision day she wrote, "I don't care that much about that specific body part, but I was hearing so much about people being so upset when they lose a breast, and I was just so confused." Nevertheless, two weeks following the surgery my mother began to confront feelings of loss over her amputated body part. In her diary she wrote, "I woke up this morning, with this real sense that losing my breast wasn't an assault on my sexuality, but on my mothering." My sister was almost five years old at the time, and my mother's breasts still represented the bond they shared when she breastfed my sister. In the hospital the Reach to

Recovery volunteer visited my mother to show her how to wear prostheses. It led her to wonder whether "there is a whole little cult of women out there who have had mastectomies." But as a large-breasted woman, she found that the heavy, uncomfortable, fake breast did not work for her. Instead she imagined a prophylactic mastectomy as the most functional way to cope with a surgically altered body. Having her other breast removed would make her feel less lopsided.

In addition to the surgery, my mother endured six months of chemotherapy in the form of 3 Adriamycin/Cytoxan, 6 Cytoxan/methotrexate, and 5FU (Fluorouracil). All her hair fell out over a two-day period. My maternal grandmother cut off the remaining chunks of hair and my father shaved the rest to make it easier for her to go bald or to wear hats and wigs. The first course of chemotherapy made her sicker than the cancer itself. So on the two-year anniversary of her first surgery, when some calcifications showed up in her right breast, rather than having a biopsy, she chose the path of least resistance. She had a simple mastectomy with a small lymph-node dissection. (Because she opted for this hastened procedure, the insurance company decided not to cover this $10,000 operation.) She perceived the second mastectomy to be worth it: "I am so much more comfortable. . . . I can go without anything in most clothes, and I don't think people really notice. If they do, so what. . . . I'm a cancer survivor. I know the big secret. I've seen death, and I've seen life, and I like life better."

Three years following two mastectomies, radiation, and chemotherapy, the breast cancer continued to metastasize in my mother's body. This time a tumor appeared in her neck. To arrest the latest cancer metamorphosis, in the summer of 1990 my mother, grandmother, sister, and I traveled three thousand miles from Los Angeles to Boston's Dana Farber Cancer Institute. At this hospital my mother opted for the experimental stem-cell bone-marrow transplant and high-dose chemotherapy. That she could afford to travel and participate in a new clinical trial makes my family's upper-middle-class privilege clear. Few women are able to take part in medical studies even in their own cities because of economic or insurance constraints. This treatment consisted of four cycles of outpatient chemotherapy. Then, after admitting her into the hospital, the doctors extracted her bone marrow and harvested it; infused her with the experimental biological GM-CSF (granulocyte macrophage-colony stimulating factor); filtered her blood to collect the stimulated bone-marrow cells; isolated her in the hospital transplant unit; and gave her a lethal dose of chemotherapy before rescuing her with reinfused filtered cells and the frozen, harvested bone marrow. The experience took my mother literally to the brink of death and back—just barely.

The emotional repercussions of this procedure left larger scars in my mom's psyche than either surgery. The following fall she reflected on the process in her diary: "I finally got it, people with cancer don't die of cancer, they die of mental illness[;] . . . they die of living with the threat of cancer coming back at any time. It's like living with a time bomb[;] . . . you can hear the ticking, but you never know if it's going to go off or not. The uncertainty is unbearable." The ticking served as an incessant reminder that she needed to continue chemotherapy treatment off and on, which she did until her death on March 9, 1992. She believed each dosage would get her closer to my sister's graduation from high school. She hoped the bomb would not go off until she helped my sister reach adulthood.

Watching my mother subject herself to these emotionally and physically debilitating procedures affected my life dramatically. I initially observed her changing body through two mastectomies, radiation, and countless chemotherapy cycles by thinking about her shifting gender identity. My mother lived purposefully without breasts and without hair on her head, and so strangers sometimes mistook her sex: people in grocery stores and restaurants would stare at her trying to determine whether she was male or female. In the early 1990s there was no national breast cancer movement, nor was there any grassroots activism in Los Angeles (where she lived), although there was the Wellness Community, where my mother became actively involved. But, in many respects, she confronted her cancer alone.

In an attempt to comprehend what she faced in public and in private I headed to the bookstore. At the time there were not a lot of breast cancer memoirs on the shelf. In fact, the first book I read, Gilda Radner's *It's Always Something,* describes the comedian's experience with ovarian cancer. But shortly thereafter I discovered poet Audre Lorde's *The Cancer Journals* and *A Burst of Light,* and I began to understand. Her moving and lucid memoir of liver metastasis gave me a sense of the multiple ways in which this disease affected my mom. She explains, "And of course cancer is political—look at how many of our comrades have died of it during the last ten years! As warriors, our job is to actively and consciously survive it for as long as possible, remembering that in order to win, the aggressor must conquer, but the resisters need only survive. Our battle is to define survival in ways that are acceptable and nourishing to us, meaning with substance and style. Substance. Our work. Style. True to our selves" (*Burst* 98–99). Lorde in particular enabled me to apprehend several key concepts, many of which my mother's healing also depended on: the need to accept rather than hide one's postmastectomy body; the desire to have agency in one's own medical treatment; the significance of examining breast cancer from a feminist perspective; and, most important, the will to survive and struggle at all cost. This last point, perhaps, was most difficult for me to accept. Watching the devastating consequences of traditional cancer pharmaceuticals often made me resent, question, and blame those drugs for ending her life prematurely.

As an African American lesbian Lorde envisioned the battle against breast cancer in a vastly different way than my mother did; her race and sexuality could not be extracted from the way she experienced her the illness just as my mother's could not. It may have been difficult for my mom to live in a body that outsiders sometimes defined as queer. Yet as a white, heterosexual, upper-middle-class woman, her altercations did not include skirmishes with a homophobic and racist medical establishment. Lorde's words enabled me to unpack these differences and acknowledge breast cancer as a political disease—one that is greatly affected by race, sexuality, gender, and class.

If my mother's breast cancer became a harrowing familial experience, her death most certainly became the defining moment of my life. Her departure forced me to confront a second mother loss. (The woman who gave birth to me abandoned me when I was thirteen; the woman whom I call my mother had entered my life shortly before my eighth birthday.) She was the only adult who shepherded me through my tumultuous teen years. Her death occurred precisely fifteen years after she entered my life. On the fifth anniversary of her death I found myself wandering through a bookstore, drinking a cup of coffee, and browsing through the pages of *Out* magazine. In it I found an interview with Susan Love and Karin Cook. By that time I had become familiar with Love's *Breast Book,* but I had not heard of Cook or her novel, *What Girls*

Learn. I immediately purchased the hardcover book and stayed up all night until I finished it. Her remarkable and moving story about two sisters on the verge of puberty whose mother dies of breast cancer riveted me. It was precisely the cathartic text I craved.

The novel's juxtaposition of Tilden and Elizabeth's menarche alongside their mama's mastectomy and chemotherapy haunted me. Its twelve-year-old protagonist, Tilden, turns to resourceful techniques like deciphering all the new words entering her vocabulary: benign, malignant, tumor, cyst, mastectomy, cancer. She found the silence in her household around the subject of her mother's illness reflected in some of these new words, which used silent consonants. And although I was ten years older than Tilden when my mom was diagnosed, my feelings resembled hers: "I lived simultaneously with the fear and hope of seeing Mama's scar," she says (102). I too was afraid to catch a glimpse of my mother's scarred body for the first time—and later I was ashamed of that fear.

I felt connected to Tilden's narration and to the author, who, at the time, was also a twenty-eight-year-old, white lesbian and a motherless daughter because of her mother's death from breast cancer. After I corresponded with her, Cook introduced me to a community of motherless daughters—many of whose mothers had also died of breast cancer. At the center of this community was another author and text: Hope Edelman and *Motherless Daughters*.[2] This *New York Times* bestseller describes the turbulent and common stages of grief affecting girls and women who lose their mothers. Edelman, a motherless daughter herself, lost her forty-two-year-old mother to breast cancer. The great need for this book grew out of increasing mortality rates for younger women, who are often younger mothers. Motherless families increasingly saturate literary history, television, and films. However, as Edelman explains in her book, their deaths are rarely discussed, the reason they died is never disclosed, and if a visual or literary text portrays grieving, it typically hastens it and quickly moves past it.

All these texts informed my decision to write about breast cancer, for I understand the deep impact literature can have on a person's experience and, in turn, the significant effect literature can have on political and public culture. The moment my maternal grandmother handed me my mother's own diaries, quoted in this preface, I began to conceive of writing about breast cancer. Lingering over her diaries motivated me to explore a larger body of women's autobiographical writing about breast cancer. I canvassed memoirs from the previous thirty years to expand my personal investment into a literary, critical, and political endeavor. The potential of this book crystallized for me when I went to a poetry reading at the 1994 "In Queery, in Theory, Indeed" conference in Iowa City. Eve Kosofsky Sedgwick and Marilyn Hacker read from their latest works, both of which detailed their then-recent struggles with breast cancer. Hearing them helped me to broaden my sense of the types of autobiographical subjects and texts available for me to consider as I worked on this project.

When I first read my mother's diaries, I discovered one metaphor in particular that struck me and stayed with me. In January 1991, during the U.S. invasion of Iraq, she wrote: "And war broke out today. It's horrible. We attacked Baghdad. The television is full of the reports. I don't know what I feel most helpless about . . . the war in the Middle East or the war in my body." This observation came at a time when she agonized over whether to discontinue chemotherapy, although she would resort to it as well as to radiation a few months later when the cancer metastasized to her bones. She fought a war in her body by allowing toxic chemicals to infiltrate her system. And she thought about her role in a war not so much for herself but for her daughters. As a feminist and a Vietnam War protester, my mother leaned toward pacifism. And yet fighting for her life catapulted her into the role of a warrior. As my family lived with a woman struggling to stay alive, military metaphors invaded our home. We knew—whether we acknowledged it or not—that, quite literally, a ticking time bomb replaced the area of her chest wall where her breasts used to be. For five years my family tried to conquer cancer.

As a writer, my mother often resorted to metaphors similar to those in many women's memoirs about the disease. Her illness existed on multiple planes; sometimes her experience seemed so unfathomable to her that she imagined it in the context of science fiction: "It's like the monster in *Alien[;]* . . . you don't see it, you hope it's gone, but you know it's there somewhere, and that someday it's going to come out and whack you in the back of the head again, and that you're going to have to mobilize all your energy and defenses to fight it again." She concentrated all her energy to fight her disease, but her amorphous cancer cells proved to be elusive and destructive.

The science-fiction and war images that penetrate my mom's diary resonate in new ways for me today as I witness yet another invasion of Iraq, this time with the knowledge that the military interventions there have increased cancer rates for civilians and soldiers alike. Consequently, it is rather ironic for me to read Nuha al-Radi's *Baghdad Diaries,* which illustrates this connection quite clearly: "Everyone seems to be dying of cancer. Every day one hears about another acquaintance or friend of a friend dying. How many more die in hospitals that one does not know? Apparently over thirty percent of Iraqis have cancer, and there are lots of kids with leukaemia. They will never lift the embargo off us" (67). Although as an artist she does not quantify her theory, in the years since her narrative was published in 1998, some researchers have begun to study the long-term effects of depleted uranium on public health. Iraqi oncologist Mona Kammas, who has studied the impact of U.S. artillery on Iraqi civilians, has proven that cancer incidence rates in southern Iraq increased fivefold and throughout the region cancer rates doubled between 1991 and 1999. In particular, after studying 667 cases of cancer she found "the increasing prevalence was most striking in cases of leukaemia, lung cancer, bronchial cancer, cancer of the bladder, skin cancer, stomach cancer for males, and breast cancer for females" (Aitken 401).[3]

Although it is too early to know for certain the relationship between these wars and the effect they will have on breast cancer incidence rates—or indeed all cancer incidence rates—I call attention to these two narratives—one personal, the other medical—to highlight the crucial relationship between bearing witness in public and reacting to those perhaps seemingly anecdotal accounts. These types of narratives indicate why it is necessary to tell one's story and how those stories can raise public awareness and effect change. And I am reminded once again of other striking parallels in my mother's diary. Her use of war metaphors—like those invoked by so many writers with breast cancer—enabled me to think about larger connections between cancer and public health in a global context. These concerns are addressed in a 2003 issue of Breast Cancer Action's newsletter in which Executive Director Barbara Brenner argues that breast cancer, like U.S. foreign policy, does not have known long-term consequences. She argues that although we may not know what will become of Iraqis exposed to carcinogenic artillery, we must "examine the root causes, so that [we can] prevent . . . cancer or keep . . .

the international situation from developing into a crisis" ("Waging" 2). This is a lesson that can be intuited from both Rachel Carson and Audre Lorde, the women whose writing frames this study—women who provide us with a vision for thinking in proactive, precautionary terms. These texts and contexts shaped this project from its conception and helped me to articulate the power that narratives can have in the world when people listen and act.

Acknowledgments

THIS BOOK GREW out of my exposure to a variety of activist and academic experiences. Feminist scholars and breast cancer activists shaped my understanding of this disease and the power of narrative. Although I learned firsthand about breast cancer by taking care of my mother when she was sick, many women have deepened my understanding of the disease in powerful ways. Women with the Breast Cancer Alliance of Greater Cincinnati, particularly Linda Heines, Grace Hinds, and Elyce Turba, and women with Cincinnati's Hands On Lesbian Health Project—Stephanie Ballard, Anne Dollins, Lycette Nelson, and Danielle Sabrese—helped me to uncover the relationship between literature and politics. In Northampton, Massachusetts, where I worked with the Pioneer Valley Breast Cancer Network to raise awareness about the precautionary principle and to open the Cancer Connection community space for people living with cancer, I met remarkable women who improved my feminist critique of mainstream breast cancer politics and who encouraged me to consider the necessity of studying the environmental aspects of cancer. I would especially like to thank Jean Colucci, Terry Gingras, Sandy Hubbard, Ginny Kendall, Chris Manter, Deb Orgera, Anne Perkins, and Jackie Walker, who sustained me emotionally and politically as I researched this project. Because the activists I have encountered over the years continue to push toward the goals laid out by people like Rachel Carson and Audre Lorde, proceeds from this book will be donated to San Francisco's Breast Cancer Action, which embodies both writers' work most closely.

Before I could begin to write about breast cancer, I needed to learn about the disease itself from a scientific perspective. The National Breast Cancer Coalition's Project Lead (Leadership, Education, and Advocacy Development) enabled me to do precisely that. For four days in July 1998 I studied intensely with some of the most committed scientists: Ben Anderson, Michelle Bennett, Leslie Bernstein, Lundy Braun, Mary-Claire

King, Bob Millikan, and Anna Wu. These researchers donated their time to teach (primarily) women with breast cancer about the biology and epidemiology of the disease, and I am extremely grateful to have been included. The knowledge I acquired there had an enormous impact on my ability to unpack the complex statistics and language of medical journal articles, which I now use in my writing and activist work. I also want to extend my thanks to Molly Mead and Margo Michaels, who ran Project Lead, as well as my Project Lead Study group—Deborah Aldridge, Anna Gottlieb, Judith Ann Hartman, Virginia Hetrick, Judith Johnston, Carrie Nelson-Hale, and Margaret Volpe—who were a vital part of this experience; their companionship sustained me long beyond Project Lead.

Outside of these activist settings, I have encountered the generosity of scholars, artists, authors, and students. I was extremely fortunate to have the opportunity to engage with many people whose creative, intellectual, and political work informed in this book. I want to thank Karin Cook, Devra Lee Davis, Diane de Lara, Ann Fonfa, Carole Gallagher, John Gofman, Linda Lear, Ellen Leopold, Baron Lerner, Matuschka, Bob Millikan, Marion Moses, Cheryl Osimo, Carolyn Raffensperger, Eve Kosofsky Sedgwick, and Sandra Steingraber for responding to my questions about their work and their politics. They all contributed tremendously, changing the way I think about breast cancer. Librarians at the following research institutions also carefully guided me through the research process at various stages of the project: at Harvard University's Schlesinger Library, Kathy Jacob, Sarah Hutcheon, Anne Engelhart, and Kathy Herrlich; at the Alan Mason Chesney Medical Archives at the John Hopkins Medical Institutions, Gerard Shorb; and at the Lear-Carson archives at Connecticut College, Laurie Deredita.

This book was first imagined among a community of women's studies students at Miami University, many of whom created activist projects on campus or produced provocative research papers about breast cancer that propelled me to think about the importance of writing about this disease. Some of these young women also had dealt with the disease in their families and wanted to find a way to express their emotions. I would especially like to thank Sherry Eggers, Danielle Kirkland, Kendra Klein, Jamie Miracle, and Chris Rouse. Their work had a particularly important role in the incipient stages of this book, as these students constantly reminded me of the relationship between intellectual endeavors and passionate political projects. Too, my drama students at Xavier University, especially John Paul Wilchek, Hayden Hawry, and Andy Kitzmiller, stimulated my ideas about this book in its earliest beginnings.

Writing *Beyond Slash, Burn, and Poison* would not have been possible without the support of many colleagues and friends who have read and responded to various ideas or drafts of this project. Their ideas and engagement with my book complicated it and enriched it in a myriad of ways. To them I would like to extend my sincerest gratitude: Alice Adams, Pat Clark, Mary Jean Corbett, Sheila Croucher, Bonnie J. Dow, Elizabeth Swanson Goldberg, C. Lee Harrington, Robert Hayashi, Maria Hernandez, Lisa Hogeland, Frank Jordan, Kate McCullough, Angelo Robinson, Jenny Spencer, Charles Spinosa, David Swain, Jill Swiencicki, Lisa B. Thompson, and Keith Tuma. At the University of Massachusetts at Amherst I was lucky to have encountered Jenny Spencer, who allowed me to be an interloper in her dissertation writing group; the support I received from that group made this book gel in important ways. At Boise State University, my writing group has been equally instrumental in helping me unify the project while simultaneously rooting for me to complete the book. I could not have finished this manuscript without the camaraderie and feedback from Leslie Durham, Janet Holmes, Michelle Payne, Tara Penry, Jacky O'Connor, and Cathy Wagner, who helped me to think through complex ideas by posing provocative questions that ultimately made this a better book. Both of my home institutions granted me financial support to help me complete this project at various stages of my work. I am grateful to Miami University for awarding me a Sinclair Dissertation Fellowship, which provided me with the financial assistance I needed to thoroughly synthesize three years of research and put it into narrative form. At Boise State University the award of a Faculty Research Associate's Program granted me a teaching reduction, which afforded me the time necessary to revise this manuscript for publication.

Beyond Slash, Burn, and Poison also benefited from the expert guidance of Leslie Mitchner. She took this project on at its earliest stages, when it was still an amorphous dissertation. With her vision, and with the help of the most engaged and useful reader's report, Leslie encouraged me to reimagine this book in profoundly important ways. It is delightful to work with such a committed editor once again.

Because this book was composed in places that were not always close to my home institution, I have relied on the support of colleagues and friends to create intellectually stimulating communities, where I also retreated from the writing process to clear my head. I could never have completed this project without them. For sustaining me with emotional and professional support I would like to thank Jon Adams, Bruce Ballenger, Ian Barnard, Ranita Chatarjee, Martin Corless-Smith, Sharon Deevey, Tam Dinh, Kim Dugan, Amy Elder, Reshmi Dutt, Jill Gill, Alvin Greenberg, Donald Hall, Tomo Hattori, Lisa Hogeland, Janet Holmes, Karen Kelley, Karen Khale, Paul Lauter, Mara Lieberman, David Martins, Bill Maruyama, Mike Mitchell, Dana Nelson, Nick Newman, Michelle Payne, Tara Penry, Jacky O'Connor, Tom Peele, Maria Pramaggiore, Ed Rabin, Aneil Rallin, Wanda Lynn Riley, Laila Shereen, Sandra Kumamoto Stanley, Kim Thompson, Lisa B. Thompson, Tricia Waddell, and Cathy Wagner.

My book could never have been conceived—let alone delivered into the world—without the consistent and constant laughing, crying, writing, reading, sharing, discussing that took place among a vital network of friends whom I have been privileged to find. These friends, who became a kind of family, deserve medals for sticking by my side through the multiple drafts of this book. I owe an enormous debt to each of them for their tremendously helpful insight into my ideas about the relationship between literature and politics. Their patience and persistence enabled me not only to think in more complicated ways about my subject but also to say it more succinctly. Their gift of engagement in all these ways is indelibly etched in my memory. I extend my never-ending love and gratitude to Elizabeth Swanson Goldberg for enduringly strengthening my ideas, my writing, my world-view through our vital conversations; Lisa Hogeland for midwifing this book; Kate McCullough for shepherding this book from the beginning; Jill Swiencicki for creating a second home for me in Chico, which was a dynamic and vibrant place to write; Lisa B. Thompson for hashing out ideas over mushy oatmeal at Sunday morning brunches; and Karen Kahle, Laila Shereen, and Tricia Waddell for sustaining me with love and kindness as I worked through this emotionally draining project.

This book is dedicated to the woman whose memory shapes everything I do, my mother, Jane Gibbons-Knopf. She was a reporter and freelance writer who, like Rose Kushner, did not live to see much of her work published. I took on this project in large part to honor her legacy as a woman who did not survive breast cancer and as a writer who kept diaries detailing her plight with the disease. My maternal grandma, Marian Newman Gibbons, engendered this book when she first gave me my mother's diaries. Her encouragement, in addition to the support of my grandpa Jim Gibbons, my paternal grandparents, Sylvia and Siggy Knopf, my father, David Knopf, and my brother, Shane Knopf, was steadfast.

While revising this manuscript, I discovered yet another way that my mother's legacy affects me. She entered my life when I was an eight-year-old girl in desperate need of a mother who would protect me and teach me about the world. Two years ago I found myself in a parallel situation; I became part of a family in which I could provide similar guidance and love to a child who needed and deserved it. Being embraced by this family has enhanced my life exponentially and in profound ways. Like Rachel Carson, I find myself struggling to find the words to describe or explain how important Murli Nagasundaram and Divy Murli are to me. Their presence has dramatically improved my writing, my teaching, and my life. I am grateful to them beyond words.

*Beyond Slash, Burn,
and Poison*

Introduction

English novelist Frances Burney wrote one of the earliest patient accounts of a mastectomy. Although most women with breast cancer in the early nineteenth century discovered their illness after the lump became visible, Burney discovered hers when she felt a small, painful swelling in her breast. The primary document, which narrates her illness, is in the form of a letter in which she couches her medical experience in legal metaphors. She envisions herself as a criminal who must submit to her "sentence" and consequently sits in wait "of a summons to execution" by the "judge" (134). It is not unique that a woman would write about her fears of an impending mastectomy; what is remarkable about Burney's writing is her memory and description of the operation itself. Because Burney lived in France at the time (1811), Dominique-Jean Larrey, Napoleon's army surgeon, performed her operation with the assistance of several nurses, doctors, and maids. Unlike a doctor's version of mastectomy, Burney's account bears witness to the somatic pain of ablation without anesthesia and without antiseptic; her surgeon gave her only "a wine cordial" to calm her nerves (136). In a letter to her family dated September 30, 1811, she describes the experience of having her right breast removed with the same kind of riveting suspense she evokes in her novels:

> When the dreadful steel was plunged into the breast—cutting through veins—arteries—flesh—nerves—I needed no injunctions not to restrain my cries. I began a scream that lasted unintermittingly during the whole time of the incision—& I almost marvel that it rings not in my Ears still! so excruciating was the agony. When the wound was made, & the instrument was withdrawn, the pain seemed undiminished, for the air that suddenly rushed into those delicate

parts . . . felt like a mass of minute but sharp & forked poniards, that were tearing the edges of the wound—but when again I felt the instrument—describing a curve—cutting against the grain, if I may so say, while the flesh resisted in a manner so forcible as to oppose & tire the hand of the operator, who was forced to change from the right to the left—then, indeed, I thought I must have expired. . . . Oh Heaven!—I then felt the Knife <rack>ling against the breast bone—scraping it!—This performed, while I yet remained in utterly speechless torture, I heard the Voice of Mr. Larr[e]y,—(all others guarded a dead silence) in a tone nearly tragic, desire every one present to pronounce if any thing more remained to be done. . . . The finger of Mr. Dubois—which I literally *felt* elevated over the wound, though I saw nothing, & though he touched nothing, so indescribably sensitive was the spot—pointed to some further requisition—& again began the scraping! (138–139)

I quote from her letter at length because it of its unprecedented significance. Even though it remained unpublished and fairly private for over 150 years, it is one of the first-known documents recording this excruciating and mutilating surgery with exacting precision. It also demonstrates a narrative style of chronicling mastectomy nonexistent in the twentieth-century texts I analyze in this book—that is, it offers the perspective of a woman conscious on the operating table rather than a woman's response to the surgery after waking up without her breast(s). On one level Burney's letter reveals the intensely personal experience of a woman witnessing the removal of her breast, although she later shared the story with her family in England. On another level her letter not only stands as a literary text but also serves as a document of medical history. Although she did not publish her story in a newspaper or a book, it eventually circulated among surgeons who gained perspective on the patient's subjectivity. Thus, Burney laid the groundwork for the tradition of testimonial intervention; women later wrote in this form with the purposeful intention of conveying their traumatic experiences with breast cancer treatment in order to alter medical practices.

To give an idea of a more typical operation at the time, that same year John and Abigail Adams's daughter, Abigail Adams Smith, also had a mastectomy. Her doctors gave her opium as an anesthetic, but unlike

Burney she neither wrote about the procedure nor survived it for very long. She died of breast cancer two years later, in 1813. (Because Burney lived until 1840, some believe that her lump was perhaps not malignant.) At a moment in history when no one had any agency in medical procedures, Burney's voice worked in an empowering way even though she felt powerless, as literary critic Julia Epstein reveals: "To write her own medical history . . . was to undertake her own surgery: to control the probe, the knife, the wound, and the blood herself; to speak for the wound's gaping unspeakableness—the woman her own surgeon, both reopening and reclosing the incisions in her own body and in the body of her writing" (82). For Burney, then, writing was a tool that assisted her in becoming empowered; and in that process she gained some agency by representing her body. Putting language to the torturous act of ablation without anesthesia, Burney took control over her recovery by controlling its narrative. Eventually those words provided the historical context for the trajectory of women's writing about mastectomy.

As one might imagine, the disfiguring and painful results of mastectomy led women to focus on that particular aspect in their writing. At the time of Burney's surgery, modern conventional medical treatments like chemotherapy and radiation did not exist. Moreover, because physicians lacked practical training on women's bodies, breast cancer often went untreated except for palliative care. In the late nineteenth century, when doctors informed the white American diarist Alice James (sister of novelist Henry James and psychologist William James) that she had a cancerous lump in her breast, they ordered no further treatment. On the occasion of her initial diagnosis she reveals, in a diary entry dated May 31, 1891, that the doctors said that "a lump I have had in one of my breasts for three months, which has given me a great deal of pain, is a tumor; that nothing can be done for me but to alleviate the pain; that it is only a question of time, etc" (231). Because she spent her life dodging various unnamed or unacknowledged illnesses, she had a unique approach to this news: she relished it. She almost reveled in the ability to label her suffering: "the lump in Alice's breast was a welcome sign, the solid emblem of a perverse kind of achievement" (Yeazell 2). Doctors managed her pain with morphine, and she occasionally considered whether she should ask her lover "for K[atherine]'s lethal dose" as she did one last time on the night before her death (James 252).

Ultimately James did not resort to suicide to cure her pain. But a diagnosis of breast cancer, understandably, led other women to contemplate such action. Forty-three years after James's death, white American feminist Charlotte Perkins Gilman ended her life instead of submitting to surgery or x-ray treatment, which she believed would enhance—rather than reduce—her suffering. In the final chapter of her autobiography she explains, "In January 1932, I discovered that I had cancer of the breast. . . . I had not the least objection to dying. But I did not propose to die of this, so I promptly bought sufficient chloroform as a substitute" (333). She feared not only the painful elements of the disease's progression but also the treatment, which to her seemed equally horrific. Other women chose similar alternative paths. When diagnosed with terminal breast cancer in 1908, white American writer Mary Austin refused to have a mastectomy or any other medical treatment. Instead she chose an unconventional method of therapy: she traveled to an Italian convent where she learned a specific form of healing prayer. A few years later, in 1912, Mohawk poet Pauline Johnson-Tekahionwake disguised her impending death from metastatic breast cancer in an autobiographical poem about war, one of the earliest writings about breast cancer by a Native Canadian writer.

These early representations of breast cancer set a precedent for characterizing it as something to fear, hide, and die of. Because most of the above-mentioned texts did not reach the public until after the authors' deaths (James's diaries were not published until 1934; Burney's letter did not appear in a book until 1975), discussions about the devastating effects of breast cancer also remained hidden. And once they found a public audience, they did not necessarily attract a readership of women with breast cancer. In each of these autobiographical texts the illness exists as one subject among many. Or it remains buried beneath the surface of larger issues the author grapples with. In addition, with the exception of Johnson-Tekahionwake's poem, these texts entrench the perspective of middle-class white women as the dominant view of the disease. During the nineteenth and early twentieth centuries medical men who examined black women tended to categorize all women of color as objects not subjects. And because women of color—historically and currently—tend to get diagnosed at a later stage of the disease, the chance for living long enough to write about breast cancer decreases. As a result, breast cancer was seen as predominantly afflicting white, middle-class women—a perception that has changed relatively little in the last century.

But much did change over the course of the twentieth century. Now women tell their stories about breast cancer on the Internet, in courts of law, in magazines, in Congress, in diaries, in doctors' offices, and on television. In the 1990s women produced poetry, plays, memoirs, films, comic books, novels, essays, and self-help manuals about breast cancer, most of which included descriptions of their own struggles with the illness. The large number of first-person accounts about breast cancer constitutes a separate subgenre of autobiography. Stories about fighting breast cancer do not always remain in the pages of books or in the privacy of hospital rooms. Women with breast cancer who join organizations like the National Breast Cancer Coalition (NBCC) and lobby on their behalf find themselves reiterating their stories in front of their congressional representatives. In fact, the NBCC advocates that women use their anecdotes to capture the attention of their legislators.[1] By appealing to their empathetic sensibilities, the theory goes, breast cancer activists can accrue support for the passage of NBCC's legislative agenda. Indeed, at its 1998 conference, then-First Lady Hillary Rodham Clinton practiced that strategy. She framed her discussion around her own familial connection to the disease by sharing a story about her mother-in-law's breast cancer. She intended that story to encourage activists to never give up fighting, just as they would never concede if it meant the life or death of a loved one. That same month she repeated portions of this story in a *Ladies' Home Journal* article to convey her support for Medicare-funded "mommograms," as she referred to them.

Beyond Slash, Burn, and Poison follows a similar method. Examining women's narratives about breast cancer, I trace the evolution of the subject from Rachel Carson's private letters to Audre Lorde's published journals, which galvanized women to take a more active role in their healthcare and which eventually mobilized women to overcome the barriers to women's agency in the medical system. The texts I explore in this book illustrate the symbiotic relationship among culture, politics, and medicine. I argue that each woman's writing on the subject had an impact and led to changes in public policy or medical practices or both. Cases of literature effecting medical or legislative change may be difficult to flesh out, but this book demonstrates how to draw some conclusions about the power of literature in the public sphere. Autobiographical prose bleeds into medical institutions and congressional offices. Perhaps because readers ascribe a truth value to a firsthand account, authors are called on to become spokespeople or activists who lobby Congress to allocate funds for cancer research. Alternately, patients who face a diagnosis of breast cancer turn to memoirs for advice, catharsis, and commiseration.

Silent Surgery?

Because Burney wrote so boldly about her breast cancer almost two hundred years ago, it may seem that she lived in a world that openly discussed medical topics and perhaps women's bodies. Although some women may have spoken openly about breast cancer with family members or medical professionals, women typically did not write about or discuss the subject in public settings. Part of the reason for the silence about women's breasts and the diseases they possibly carry has to do with the varied and conflicting cultural meanings assigned to breasts. Even prior to the obsession of the mass media in the United States with the sexual significance of breasts, women learned at an early age to revere (and sometimes to reveal) their breasts. Consequently, breast cancer is both a dreaded and a gendered disease for women. A breast gives life when mothers feed their children. A breast supplies women with sexual pleasure. And that same breast can be invaded by cancer cells that threaten the lives of women and mothers.

A cancerous breast tumor threatens the life not only of the woman/mother but of her nuclear family as well. Fear of such tumors developed during the Victorian era, when the breast—in a literal and a metaphorical sense—represented the hearth of the family. Ellen Leopold explains that the breast's iconic power reminded a woman to "put the needs of others before her own. Any pleasure a woman might take in her own body or her own life was deemed to be inconsequential to the culture, a secondary effect, derived from the pleasure she gave to others. What did matter was the preservation of family life. Inescapably, breast cancer put this at risk" (*A Darker* 31). Leopold's assessment reveals why the heteronormative familial structure contributed to harboring a woman's illness as a secret. In the nineteenth-century United States, once people interpreted breast cancer as a disease that could destroy the nuclear family, it became necessary for secrecy to prevail inside the domestic sphere.

The rise of surgery grew out of the secrecy that surrounded breast cancer and protected the family. Unlike Burney, a woman typically knew that something was wrong with her body once she saw the tumor protruding from her breast, often accompanied by symptoms like bleeding nipples and severe pain. In this context, removal of the breast offered the woman palliative treatment. Once the woman recovered from her mastectomy, Leopold explains, "she could reenter society or play a more active role in domestic life without drawing attention to her physical loss. While this may have preserved her sense of privacy and restored some sense of normalcy, it implicitly placed a higher value on the social denial of the disease than on the private need to unburden oneself. A woman with breast cancer, in other words, soon discovered that surgery itself created some disturbing conflicts" (*A Darker* 67).

The cultural burden that the breast bears is important to consider, but breast cancer existed long before any Victorian codes of morality limited public discussion of women's bodies. Although doctors have practiced surgery as a remedy for breast cancer since antiquity, the method that unremittingly eroded women's agency in their healthcare in the twentieth century was first used during the Enlightenment, when Benjamin Bell established the need for expediency between diagnosis and surgery; as a result, determining whether a tumor was malignant merged with surgical treatment. In consequence women would not know their diagnosis or prognosis until both the mastectomy and the biopsy were completed.[2] Coupling Bell's procedure with Bernhard Perilhe's theories, which argued for the removal of the pectoral muscles in addition to the breast, one finds the roots of what would become known as the Halsted radical mastectomy. Through the convergence of these two procedures women would be dismissed when it came to making decisions about treating their bodies. This inadvertent, systematic silencing of women endured until the late twentieth century. These procedures were not devised as some malicious way to torture women or to repress their voices. However, the way in which these practices became codified and remained unquestioned over the course of two centuries led to precisely this result.

Making breast surgery standard during the eighteenth century was more difficult than it later became, as Burney's letter attests, because no anesthetics or antiseptics existed. But Burney benefited from the Napoleonic wars, which led to the training of an enormous number of surgeons on the battlefield; although the bodies they practiced on were male, these surgeons used the opportunity to refine their skills because the cadavers provided them with an opportunity to increase their knowledge of human anatomy. However, as one might expect, ablation became a viable treatment for breast cancer only after the development of surgical anesthesia in 1846. And it became conventional only with the invention of a wound antiseptic in 1877. These pivotal discoveries, made at a time when doctors acquired and practiced specialties, changed the face of surgical medicine in general and the treatment of breast cancer more particularly.

The medical inventions that made surgery safer and cleaner enabled William Stewart Halsted to study the effectiveness of regularly removing the pectoral muscles in all mastectomies. As a professor of surgery at the Johns Hopkins College of Medicine, he made recommendations about mastectomy that became institutionalized by his students, who later worked in the field; publication of his ideas in medical journals further implanted his beliefs and practices. In order to assist the establishment of his version of the mastectomy, Halsted laid out the specific criteria for the operation: "*The pectoralis major muscle, entire or all except its clavicular portion, should be excised in every case of cancer of the breast. . . . The suspected tissues should be removed in one piece lest the wound become infected by the division of tissues invaded by the disease, or of lymphatic vessels containing cancer cells, and because shreds or pieces of cancerous tissue might be readily overlooked in a piecemeal extirpation*" (11; emphasis in original). Halsted explained his procedure with precision. He also ensured that surgeons would have a lucid picture of the operation from his words and from his diagrams (Figure 1).

Halsted feared the spread of cancer cells through the local lymph nodes so he rationalized that women benefited from the removal of extensive quantities of muscle, tissue, and cells. To support his theory, epidemiologists began to track mortality and incidence rates for breast cancer around the turn of the century. Those statistics reinforced the early-twentieth-century belief that a woman could choose only between a Halsted radical mastectomy and death. Largely because the epidemiological data seemed to confirm the success of Halsted radical mastec-

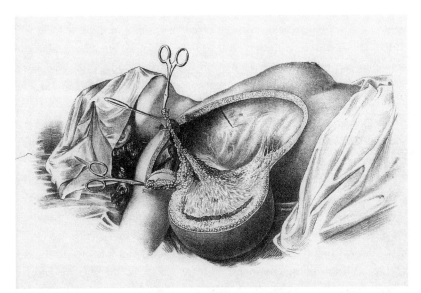

1. Illustration of a Halsted radical mastectomy. Courtesy, The Alan Mason Chesney Medical Archives of the Johns Hopkins Medical Institutions.

tomies, this practice remained unchallenged until First Lady Betty Ford's operation in 1974 opened up the debates to a wide public audience. Although surgeons like the Cleveland Clinic's George Crile Jr. had risked their professional standing to critique some of the compulsory surgical and oncological practices for a lay audience, a woman could not speak publicly about her illness using the words *breast* and *cancer* in the same sentence. The publicity of the then–first lady's surgery set the stage for Crile and the pioneering breast cancer activist Rose Kushner to make breast cancer's outmoded treatment history.

As a surgeon and a writer Crile began to question the efficacy of radical surgery in the mainstream mass media in ways that laid the foundation for women to eventually participate in the debate. As early as 1955, as Barron Lerner explains, Crile "completely stopped performing the classic Halsted radical mastectomy, likely becoming the only surgeon in the United States to have done so" (*Breast Cancer* 104). Instead he performed one of three procedures, depending on the pathology of the tumor: a simple mastectomy (removal of the breast), a partial mastectomy (which later became known as a lumpectomy), or a modified radical mastectomy, which left the chest wall undisturbed. That same year, in the pages of *Life* magazine, Crile criticized his colleagues for scaring the public about cancer and its typical healing regimen. The charged article appeared alongside perspectives from surgeons and advocates associated with organizations such as the American Cancer Society (ACS), the American Medical Association (AMA), the National Cancer Institute (NCI), and the American College of Surgeons, all of which called his medical ethics into question for revealing his theories about cancer to a lay audience.[3]

As this debate over breast cancer surgery grew, one aspect of Crile's critique in particular likely worried surgeons. He disclosed the financial rewards of surgery that privileged the Halsted: surgeons billed for their work based on how much of the body they cut away. Confronted with this uniform practice, he stated, "I knew that . . . sooner or later in the U.S.A., in spite of the temptation to over-operate that fee-for-service medicine gave, the public would become informed and seek out surgeons who would not unnecessarily mutilate them. Then everyone would have to agree that the radical mastectomy was obsolete" (*Way* 329). Making the lucrative incentive for doctors to continue radical mastectomy public triggered a lifelong struggle among Crile, other surgeons, and the ACS.

Crile furthered his medical-political agenda to inform his patients when he authored two pivotal books: *Cancer and Common Sense* (1955) and, after he retired, *What Women Should Know about the Breast Cancer Controversy* (1973). Both were unique in medical history because he wrote for lay readers. His books empowered patients to understand treatment options and to make their own choices about their bodies. The details that he shared with a wide audience alarmed his colleagues. Before he presented his findings to the public, doctors rarely informed their patients of alternative surgical options or complementary treatment possibilities. Those patients who questioned their physicians or pursued other options found it difficult to oppose both their doctors and the disease simultaneously. Although many surgeons relied on dense language and a discipline that obscured its practices, Crile exposed that rhetoric, the procedures, and their limitations to the general public. His clinically supported theories challenged the established methods of treating women with breast cancer by advocating breast-conserving surgeries. Eventually women with breast cancer joined him in publicly presenting their first-hand accounts about the trauma of Halsted radical mastectomies or the exhilaration of having agency in the healthcare decision-making process.

Over the course of twenty years Crile also published several condemnations of the Halsted in medical journals. However, he waited until he retired to share the bulk of his research on breast cancer with a mass public because he worried about being accused "of publicizing my beliefs to increase my practice" (*What Women* 12). Much of his motivation for writing for lay readers came from his sincere empathy for his patients, most notably his deceased wife, Jane Halle Crile. He demonstrated his compassion by weaving some of her story into his book about breast cancer in order to break down some of the well-established barriers between doctors and patients. In her memory he divulged his primary findings to clarify the misinterpretations in mass-media reporting about breast cancer surgery: "In the past five years I have also become convinced that in properly selected cases, equivalent results can be obtained by even simpler operations in which only a part of the breast is removed. I have reported our results with partial mastectomy at the Cleveland Clinic in scientific papers and have quoted the reported results of surgeons in England and Scandinavia who have used similar treatment with good results; these reports have in turn been made public in women's magazines, where they have sometimes been misunderstood" (*What Women* 11). His data about partial mastectomy provided yet another choice for women depending on the size of the lump and the likelihood of metastasis: in a partial mastectomy only the cancerous lump is removed; the rest of the breast remains intact with only a small scar.

Yet his data on new findings continued to be misconstrued, sometimes by his peers and sometimes by the media; his colleagues met the publicness of his research and writing with hostility. For instance, during the onslaught of publicity surrounding Ford's and Happy Rockefeller's (different) surgeries, sometimes the mass media incorrectly reported medical research. Stories about mastectomy tended not to present crucial facts about different stages and types of breast cancer that could dictate surgical options. When the media invoked Crile's name in these stories, he could not control how they presented his research to the public. Women reading *Good Housekeeping* did not necessarily have the tools to differentiate surgical opinions and options.

Ultimately Crile found a public, pedagogic platform to teach women about choices they could make when confronted with a breast cancer diagnosis. He empowered his patients to such an extent that one woman, Rosamond Campion, wrote a memoir about the validation she felt because she chose her own surgery. Crile argues that her book "and the discussion it provoked on television . . . did more to bring the breast cancer controversy to the attention of the public than anything else" (*What Women* 13). He claims her memoir helped him to disseminate his message. However, because Campion's book was written under a pseudonym (her name was Babette Rosamond) and because the disease was disguised in the book's title, *The Invisible Worm*, she did not galvanize the public in nearly the same way that Ford, Kushner, and Lorde later did when they openly discussed their bodies and their illness using explicit language. If Campion's work had been less obscured by metaphorical images and a veiled identity, perhaps the debate would have attracted a larger and more sustained following, and the first lady's surgeon might have advised her that she could choose a less mutilating surgery. Nevertheless, the reliance of both Crile and Campion on the feminist rhetoric of choice, which became dominant in the burgeoning second-wave feminist movement, provided a context and a platform for the critiques later launched by Lorde and Kushner.

Perhaps if other physicians had communicated openly with their patients, Ford's surgeon might have shared Pittsburgh surgeon Bernard Fisher's early results from the first randomized clinical trial comparing the Halsted radical mastectomy to a simple (total) mastectomy. (In the United States a treatment modality gains acceptance through randomized clinical trials.) In 1979, Fisher released the first findings to indicate "no survival advantage to radical mastectomy" (Lerner, *Breast Cancer*, 225). Lerner explains that "the most revolutionary aspect of Bernard Fisher's findings was that failure to treat the axillary lymph nodes had no effect on survival from breast cancer. It was the intricate dissection and removal of all accessible lymph nodes along with the rooting out of as much local cancer as possible, that had been the basis of Halsted's theories" (*Breast Cancer* 238). Although the work of Fisher, Crile, and other surgeons effectively challenged and eventually changed the course of breast cancer surgical—and later adjuvant—treatment, the role of women's increasing involvement in these public debates and in private consultation with their doctors cannot be underestimated.

TAKING BACK THE BODY

Mastectomy and hysterectomy share a history of surgical practices and of women's relative silence about the subject. Leopold compares these two procedures with this perspective in mind: "Both evolved, over time, from a procedure that removed a single organ to one that included the resection of a variety of other muscles, tissue, glands, or organs. In the case of hysterectomy, this might include the ovaries, vagina, or cervix as well as pelvic lymph nodes and other tissues" (*A Darker* 206). Like mastectomy, the hysterectomy, from its origin in the nineteenth century, was performed to eliminate a variety of reproductive cancers. But this invisible surgery is set apart because it emerged as an operation that could theoretically counteract any number of female complaints, such as endometriosis, prolapsed uterus, backache, menstrual cramps, and fibroid tumors. Moreover, by the 1970s some gynecological surgeons believed that the hysterectomy could be used as a prophylactic to prevent cancer, control fertility, and terminate menstruation. As this list expanded so too did women's increasing concern that the hysterectomy had become a catch-all and an excuse to overoperate on women.

The general practice of not discussing a woman's medical treatment with her carried over into this gendered surgery as well. Although women's uteruses are not fetishized the same way that their breasts are and although this body part lies hidden from public view, many of the side effects of a hysterectomy were quite debilitating, including the late-nineteenth- and early-twentieth-century proscriptions about not discussing women's bodies or health. According to Leopold, "Besides the abrupt loss of fertility that could never be reversed, there were several serious health problems that could develop. These included urinary disorders, loss of bone density, loss of protection against heart disease brought on by premature menopause, loss of sexual desire, and joint aches and pains. But physicians had not warned their patients of any of these possibilities. They had told them of no risks or side effects. This made it much harder for women to describe or seek some kind of recognition for symptoms not acknowledged by the doctors they had trusted so completely" (*A Darker* 209). Thus private and public silence ensued about the psychological and physiological remnants of this surgical abstraction.

The striking similarities between the types of surgery used to extract cancer of the breast and those used to treat cancer of the uterus caused many women and doctors to lump all the various reproductive cancers into one category. When writers did venture into the mainstream media to educate women about these procedures, they were sometimes grouped together, as Kirsten Gardner describes: "The literature about women and cancer, especially in the pre-1950 popular press, often combined information about all female cancers. Until the 1940s 'reproductive cancers' that included cancers of the cervix, ovary, and uterus, caused more death for more women than breast cancer. Unlike today, the fear of breast cancer was no more significant than the fear of 'generative organ cancers.' Women often learned about these four cancers at the same time and from the same source, thereby perceiving 'female cancers' as a single category" (8–9). These magazine articles lifted some of the silences around cancer, but still the language often veiled the subject by using imprecise words or by feeding into women's fears of these dreaded diseases and the methods used to treat them.

As routinized hysterectomy gained favor with the medical community, so, too, did women's vocal and critical responses to it. Ann Dally explains that "gradually techniques improved and, during the twentieth century, hysterectomy became enormously popular. It became safer, increased in popularity and replaced ovariotomy [or oophorectomy] as a common operation that could be done even when the problem was vague or psychiatric" (220). At the same time, because of the increasing relative safety of the procedure "it was being performed on so many women that, at least in the United States, there were now more deaths from hysterectomy than from cancer of the womb" (221). Statistics like these effectively galvanized medical, political, and lay critics of this overused procedure to try to decrease the frequency with which gynecologists relied on it. Around the same time that women began to speak out about and organize around breast cancer, in the late 1970s, women gathered as witnesses before Congress to testify about the overuse of hysterectomies, particularly in cases where it was employed to regulate fertility or to prevent cancer. Given that "of the 725,000 hysterectomies performed in 1975, only twenty per cent could be justified as treatment for cancer or other life-threatening disorders," women who challenged the widespread use of this procedure were able to make a convincing case before their legislators (Dally 222–223).

Organizing around the issue of hysterectomy made sense within the context of the burgeoning women's health movement. Those who worked in this facet of the feminist movement focused on helping women obtain medical attention free from discrimination and assisted women in achieving agency in their healthcare.[4] Many of these activists also compiled and wrote books in which they carefully documented these pressing health and illness concerns. Books like Claudia Dreifus's *Seizing Our Bodies*, Cynthia Cooke and Susan Dworkin's *The Ms. Guide to a Woman's Health*, Sheryl Burt Ruzek's *The Women's Health Movement*, and Elizabeth Fee's *The Politics of Sex in Medicine* pinpointed obstacles facing women in the medical system.[5] Perhaps the most famous text of this period was the Boston Women's Health Book Collective's *Our Bodies, Ourselves*. Its first edition, which, like most publications coming out of the women's health movement, centered on white women's health, further embedded that model in the medical establishment.[6]

Although breast cancer appears in these books, the authors do not make it a primary concern. Most of the women active in groups like the Boston Women's Health Book Collective were young, and consequently they focused, at least initially, on issues connected to reproductive health. In the pre– and post–*Roe v. Wade* climate, the primarily white, working- and middle-class women creating what would become *Our Bodies, Ourselves* found ways to educate themselves about and to teach others how to wrest control of their bodies away from medical doctors and to place that power in their own hands. Thus, hysterectomy emerged as a prominent subject for the women's health movement because of the natural link between fertility and sterility as well as because of the desire to maintain control over one's own body—issues that affected young women in greater numbers than did women's cancers or heart disease. However, although women certainly faced physiological and psychological issues post-hysterectomy and although women also had to contend with the silence historically surrounding such a procedure, they did not tend to author memoirs about their sense of loss or their anger about what had been done to their bodies. Moreover, arguably, because there were no celebrities as powerful and as famous as the first lady of the United States leading the effort to speak out against the overuse of hysterectomies and because the uterus is not hypersexualized the way breasts are, the debate surrounding the overzealous use of hysterectomies did not attract the same level of media attention that breast cancer did.

Even though the first women to publicly speak about breast cancer—both famous women like Ford and activists like Kushner—did so in a moment that was made possible by the awareness created in the media by the women's liberation and women's health movements, the issues and their spokespeople were not immediately well understood or known. Maintaining control over one's body—whether through Pap smears or breast self-exam—did not necessarily cover the same demographics as cancer did. Therefore, as Sandra Morgen explains, "the first edition of Our Bodies, Ourselves made only brief references to breast, cervical, or uterine cancers," but its first mainstream edition, published in 1973, includes several pages on these diseases (143). It took ten more years for an edition to cover all the major illnesses that women face with material specific to women's needs. Thus, although ultimately during the 1970s women began to speak out publicly about their bodies and their health, the discussion took different forms depending on the issue as well as on whom it affected and how it affected them. And, because of the work of these women, breast cancer crept into public discourse with increasing frequency and alacrity.

PUBLICIZING CANCER

The United States during the 1970s witnessed such a wide variety of feminist activism surrounding women's equality and women's bodies it seemed as if it were the first time women had banded together to raise awareness about issues like breast cancer. But in fact women began speaking out about cancer, in all its various forms, during the first part of the twentieth century; in this previous incarnation raising awareness about cancer did not require women to separate the various reproductive diseases. When the ACS (originally named the American Society for the Control of Cancer) formed in 1913, it was dedicated to teaching the public about cancer prevention and treatment. Twenty-two years later, and one year prior to the formation of the NCI, the agency inaugurated a program called the Women's Field Army. The mainly white, middle-class housewives dressed in military-style uniforms and carried promotional posters. As James Patterson describes it, "Posters and handbills listed Eleanor Roosevelt and other national figures as honorary supporters and featured the [American Society for the Control of Cancer's] symbol, a flaming sword that glowed with spirit and determination. 'There SHALL be light!' these proclaimed: 'ENLIST IN WOMEN'S FIELD ARMY!' Thus armed, the officers hoped to build an army of foot soldiers who would carry the message of early detection and medical intervention into every home in the land" (122).

The charged rhetoric the Women's Field Army used in its poster campaign mirrored the language of war, but it also made clear that this was a new subject for public discourse. As the Women's Field Army embarked on its door-to-door campaign to instruct women about cancer of the breast and uterus, it ended the silences surrounding those subjects. The volunteers encouraged women to get annual pelvic examinations, despite the fact that women in the 1930s felt uncomfortable going to predominantly male gynecologists to have their private parts examined.

In an interesting example of coalition politics, over two million women joined the Women's Field Army through clubs like the Young Women's Christian Association, the Associated Women of the American Farm Bureau Federation, the National Association of Colored Women, and the Jewish women's organization Hadassah. Leslie Reagan describes how the volunteers "represented ethnically and racially diverse populations" and created programs "that included not only well-to-do and middle-class women but working-class women as well" (1780). Although the Women's Field Army made attempts to collaborate with other ladies' organizations that it believed would help spread the message of examination, detection, and treatment while lessening some of the fears women felt about the disease, most of the white, middle-class women running the organization did not effectively leave behind their segregated lives as they reached out to communities of color and poor communities. Perhaps conflicting perceptions of the disease also thwarted their efforts. Lerner explains some of these considerations: "In contrast to diseases such as tuberculosis, which predominated among the poor, cancer was seen as a disease that affected all women. Indeed, in the case of breast cancer, the limited data indicating that morbidity and mortality from the disease were higher among the wealthy may have discouraged targeted publicity efforts in poor and minority neighbor-hoods" (*Breast Cancer* 47).

Thus, albeit inadvertently, the Women's Field Army's work rein-forced the perception that breast cancer is a disease of affluence. The problem with this perception is that even during the time of the Women's Field Army's operation, statistics indicated that poor women had higher mortality rates than their wealthier counterparts, likely because their cases were not diagnosed until the disease was at a later stage (Kraus and Oppenheim, cited in Lerner, *Breast Cancer*). The Women's Field Army had the potential to make its mission much more public and thereby to make a difference in rural and urban areas, where poorer women resided. But, according to Lerner, this enormous potential was not fully realized: "Whereas only 10 percent of whites had never heard of the cancer soci-ety, this figure reached 33 percent among African Americans" (*Breast Cancer* 47). Unfortunately, neither the ACS nor the Women's Field Army honed in on the ways in which race, class, and gender overlapped in the health needs of women. Therefore, when investigating specifically gendered aspects of cancer, studies—as was common practice for the time—did not differentiate in terms of race or class to discern the par-ticular types of outreach or treatment that might be needed in various communities.

The Women's Field Army also did not counter a 1935 medical re-port that declared, "Cancer of the breast is the penalty women pay for failing to bear and . . . nurse children" (quoted in L. Reagan 1784). The report revealed a universalized blame-the-victim mentality aimed at women who could not or chose not to have children. As Reagan sug-gests, this study blamed women "for their failure to conform to gender norms" (1784). Attributing a higher incidence of breast cancer to women without children not only complicated and compromised women's rou-tine healthcare practices (some women believed that if they had children and nursed them, they would protect themselves from gynecological cancers and therefore did not need regular checkup visits with their doc-tors) but also suggested that women had to succumb to their biological destiny as wives and mothers. The Women's Field Army contributed to this naturalizing of women's caretaking roles by "reinforc[ing] the idea that a woman was responsible for her entire community as well as herself and her family. In addition to educating women about their own cancer risk, women's organizations played a crucial role in raising money for cancer institutions, research, and the training of physicians and technicians" (L. Reagan 1785). As Reagan suggests, in many respects the Women's Field Army was hardly revolutionary or liberating. Rather, it expected women to function as caretakers in the public and the private sphere—for their own families and for everyone's family—even while it educated women about the various types of cancer that affected their bodies and jeopardized their families.

Accompanying the community educational networks of the Women's Field Army in the 1930s and 1940s were an increasing number of women's narratives about breast cancer printed in magazines. Although such reports first emerged in women's magazines during the 1910s, these "tell-all tales," as Patterson calls them, appeared with increased frequency at the same moment that the Women's Field Army gained momentum. According to Patterson, "Such stories were printed primarily in health-oriented publications such as *Hygeia*, the AMA's general circulation magazine, until the late 1940s and 1950s" (149). Women who had recovered from the disease also published their tales of hope in periodicals such as *Good Housekeeping* and the *Ladies' Home Journal.* These articles shared a focus on each woman's individual story and an undercurrent that suggested the urgent need to break the silence about discussing breast cancer in public places. The dominant message of these autobiographical accounts maintained the importance of following traditional medical guidelines of examination and treatment. However, like the Women's Field Army, these articles often addressed the same white, middle-class audience that the author herself belonged to. Those who could not afford extras like magazines, who were illiterate, or whose first language was not English would not read about self-examination or about surgical controversies as each became a subject in the media.

The public pedagogical work of doctors like Crile, which opened up the discourse about breast cancer in magazines and on television—especially as more households acquired subscriptions and television sets—was in large part dependent on cultural and political changes somewhat external to the subject of healthcare. As the various feminist and civil rights movements altered the consciousness of Americans, many activists learned their tactics and strategies from watching and reading about the strides made by those movements. Questioning the authority of politicians who challenged segregation laws or later the push to pass the Equal Rights Amendment could be applied to the ways in which women questioned their physicians' practices. As doctors and women pushed the subject of breast cancer further into the mainstream public media, the subject began to permeate arenas not targeted primarily toward a white, middle-class audience. In African American magazines such as *Ebony* and *Essence,* women—and sometimes men—with breast cancer told their stories about detection and treatment while simultaneously demystifying some of the stereotypes about who gets breast cancer and what happens postdiagnosis.

Although most features focused on average people, once celebrities came forward and shared their experiences with breast cancer, a larger audience was reached. Most remarkable was Shirley Temple Black's story in *McCall's* magazine about the importance of choosing one's own surgery. And once the first lady stepped forward, a greater number of celebrities and individuals shared their stories in the mainstream media. Although Ford was a wealthy, white celebrity like Black, her disclosure led to famous African American women such as singer Minnie Ripperton addressing a distinctly African American audience in much the same vein. Particularizing her story for black women with the help of *Ebony* magazine (Lucas), Ripperton could convey the same messages as Ford but to people in the African American community who needed to see themselves represented in this narrative about caring for one's body and one's health.

Housewives and celebrities alike helped to increase public awareness about breast cancer by reaching out to women individually and trying to alter their perceptions about and practices in taking care of their bodies. Wealthy white philanthropist Mary Lasker moved beyond the realm of narrative to increase awareness by raising money and shaping public policy. Although her fortune ironically came from her husband's efforts to encourage women to smoke Lucky Strike cigarettes during the early part of the twentieth century, by the 1940s she was determined to raise money for cancer research. Combining public-relations strategies with business fundraising tactics, she helped the ACS to capitalize on magazine articles about cancer to attract thousands of dollars in donations. After twenty years of lobbying, Lasker, along with two leading doctors, stepped up her cause with a new strategy aimed at politicians, doctors, and citizens simultaneously. Placing a full-page ad in the *New York Times* on December 9, 1969, they pleaded, "Mr. Nixon You Can Cure Cancer" (quoted in Patterson 248). According to Samuel Epstein, Lasker goaded the president and aroused citizens to join her in a letter-writing campaign "to pressure Congress to accept" recommendations to "create a National Cancer Program, with vastly expanded funds and an autonomous NCI" (289).[7] This tremendously effective publicity campaign persuaded President Richard Nixon to promise a cure in his 1971 State of the Union address. Such publicity eventually became important in laying the foundation for the work that Ford would do to increase public discourse about breast cancer three years later.

FROM THE PERSONAL TO THE HISTORICAL

According to 2002 data from the NCI's Surveillance, Epidemiology, and End Results Program, "breast cancer ranks first as the cause of death for women age 20 to 59 years" among all racial groups (Jemal et al. 35). However, as has been the case for the past few decades, African American women have the highest incidence of and mortality rates for cancer in general and for cancer of the breast and lung specifically. Breast cancer mortality rates decreased in the general female population almost 3.5 percent since 1995, and "breast cancer mortality declined in every age group except African-American women, age 75 and older" (Jemal et al. 35). Cancer incidence decreased in most ethnic groups, except for Asian/Pacific Islanders and American Indians, for whom the rates remained relatively stable. Moreover, "the mortality rate from cancer is about 33 percent higher in African Americans than among whites, and more than twice as high as cancer death rates in Asian/Pacific Islanders, American Indians, and Hispanics" (Jemal et al. 37). Although heart disease kills more women annually—373,575 women died of heart disease as opposed to 41,144 who died of breast cancer in 1999—it is the leading cause of death only for women over the age of eighty; in contradistinction breast cancer strikes at earlier ages with more lethal results (Jemal et al. 34).

As a woman whose mother died of breast cancer when she was only forty-nine, I am struck by this last statistic for personal reasons. It tugs at my emotional center because I know so many motherless daughters who often take on this new identity as a result of their mother's death from breast cancer. Since the rise of the feminist movement, many women who have chosen to pursue careers have also waited to have their children. Such lifestyle choices have implications for a woman's relative risk of being diagnosed with breast cancer; lifetime exposure to estrogen increases the later a woman has her children or if she bears no children. (Early menarche and late menopause also contribute to estrogen production.) And if a woman has children at a later stage in life and then dies from breast cancer, her children may be young when they are left motherless.

These are my personal concerns. But there are political reasons for my desire to focus on a historical examination of women's writing about breast cancer in the United States. For me, it is impossible to extract my personal motivation from my political actions, for while a woman's choices about when—or whether—to have children may alter the likelihood of her acquiring breast cancer, so too can environmental carcinogens that mimic estrogens, or xenoestrogens. And yet as writers like Carson and Lorde elucidate, many would still like to dampen awareness about environmental pollution and its relationship to cancer rates. Zillah Eisenstein puts it best when she teases out the necessary relationship between the personal and the political: "What part of the personal is not political? Is the political personal in the same fashion that the personal is political? Liberal individualism begins with the notion of privacy and the division between politics and the self. This becomes more true as the dominant discourse of neoliberalism—which emphasizes individual responsibility and favors corporate over government investment in formerly public domains—takes hold. People think more of the self, less of the public; more of the personal, less of the political; more of the self-help and less of governmental assistance; more of genes and less of environments" (139). The second-wave feminist dictum "the personal is political" has been diluted in certain public settings: the radical shift from raising one's consciousness to working in a progressive political movement has ceased at this particular historical moment—a moment when women declare in television commercials that they are "Remi-feminists" because they are savvy consumers who take "alternative" soy menopause supplements (instead of potentially carcinogenic estrogen),[8] a moment when the personal has all but squashed the political, a moment when public confessions or "Aha!" experiences on *Oprah* stand in for the more radical activism of second-wave feminism.

The dominant discourse about breast cancer certainly falls into these traps. The party line offers two types of causative narratives: family history and lifestyle choices.[9] If a woman believes that she has a genetic link to the disease because many other women in her family have breast cancer, then she cannot control it. If a woman eats a high-fat diet and later discovers that she has breast cancer, she is to blame. In both these cases the woman is encouraged to take responsibility to control her potential risk factors. Either she can change her diet (despite the fact that the environmental toxins in the fat she eats, not merely the fat in her body, might be the cause of cancer), or she can be genetically tested; if the genetic-test results are positive, she can have an oophorectomy or a prophylactic bilateral mastectomy (which, because the disease is systemic, would not decrease her likelihood of acquiring it) or she can take tamoxifen (and possibly find herself with uterine cancer—which has an even higher mortality rate than breast cancer). These are some of the options available if women relegate the personal to the private realm.

In this book I highlight women who wrote about their breast cancer and resisted the impulse to contain breast cancer in an apolitical, private space, for doing so contributes to blaming the victim, which saturates the mass-media representations of the disease. As Dorothy Nelkin and Sander Gilman explain, "Attributing cancer to lifestyle has popular appeal because it appears to enhance individual control over the disease without threatening social or political institutions" (372). By presenting a history of women who struggled to play an active role in their healing process and whose stories about that experience taught other women how to do the same, I demonstrate the importance of merging the personal with the political. Illustrating some of the ways in which women's public writing has helped to redirect the impetus to blame women, I look for answers in the larger systemic and institutional forces that they wrestled with. Each of the women in this book, in her own way, found a method of erasing some of the silence around breast cancer—the subject itself, the treatment, or hazards in the environment that might cause it.

Although many women have written about breast cancer in the United States since the 1970s, most of them have been white, middle-class, and heterosexual, and many have been Ashkenazi Jews. Confronting the layered oppressive forces in medical settings was not a priority for these women, whose white privilege sheltered them from having to think about the double or triple burdens that women of color, lesbians, and poor women carry. But a few women did intervene to counter not only the silencing of breast cancer but also the sexism, racism, classism, and homophobia in the medical establishment. With respect to breast cancer, Lorde most notably took on that role, as I discuss in Chapter Four.

In part I am interested in the overlapping relationship between women's writing about breast cancer and political gains won by feminist activists working for progressive change in the arena of healthcare. Therefore, to a certain extent this book examines the didactic effects of cultural texts. Because this project is a historical examination of breast cancer as it shifted from a private subject to a public subject, I include writers based upon their impact on the shaping of breast cancer awareness as well as on changing dominant treatment modalities and public policies from the 1960s to the 1980s. Organized chronologically, the book analyzes writings by Carson, Ford, Kushner, and Lorde as both political and literary documents; this method allows me to explore the impact of women's public witness both on the formation of breast cancer legislation and on the emerging subgenre of breast cancer literature. I argue that changes in medical practice and public policy are linked to these textual interventions.

Chapter One begins by offering a sense of what the climate was like for a woman with breast cancer before the subject became appropriate for public discourse. By exploring Rachel Carson's private letters to friends and doctors, I demonstrate the various constraints facing women—particularly those in the public eye—who felt compelled to hide their disease. Although the public did not read her letters at the time, her scientific writing and speaking challenged public policy that left carcinogenic materials unregulated in the environment. When examined together, her private and public writings paint a portrait of the tension between the treatment of breast cancer and environmental toxins. Ironically, Carson's *Silent Spring* and her congressional testimony led to changes in public policy that likely had a dramatic effect on cancer incidence rates more generally.

When First Lady Betty Ford went public with her breast cancer diagnosis in 1974, only eleven years after Carson's death, breast cancer became a subject that could be debated in the public sphere. Chapter Two traces this development through mass-media representations of Ford as well as through her autobiographical writing. Her public confession, which was in many ways enabled by a burgeoning feminist movement, became a precedent for speaking about breast cancer in public. For many women her story revealed a tragic, common practice. All women, including Ford, signed a mastectomy consent form on entering the hospital for a biopsy, and doing so kept them from knowing whether they would wake up with or without a breast. Moreover, the only sanctioned surgery—a Halsted radical mastectomy—required the removal of the pectoral muscles, the chest wall, and most of the lymph nodes under the woman's adjoining arm. No medical evidence supported this outdated and barbaric surgery, which remained entrenched in U.S. hospitals. Ford's story not only alerted women to this fact but also challenged women to gain some agency in their healthcare.

Rose Kushner capitalized on Ford's lack of agency in the navigation of her healthcare. In Chapter Three I illustrate how Kushner used her skills as a journalist to make breast cancer a public and a political subject. From a political perspective this chapter provides the most clear-cut example of how writing influences public policy and changes medical practice. I document this progression by showing how the media spectacle surrounding the first lady's surgery created a platform from which Kushner worked to eradicate the Halsted radical mastectomy and to allow women to separate the biopsy from the surgical procedure. To accomplish these tasks she wrote the first self-help manual for women with breast cancer, based on her experience with the illness, and she testified before Congress on the subject.

In Chapter Four I highlight the remarkable differences made in one woman's life by the changes Kushner facilitated. However, one of the silences that neither Kushner nor Ford broke was the silence surrounding the fact that breast cancer mortality rates for women of color and poor women were dramatically higher than for white, middle-class women. Although women increasingly went public with their illness, those who did established a white, middle-class association with the disease. Through the writing of Audre Lorde, my book concludes by magnifying the particular concerns that one black lesbian had when she encountered the traditional medical establishment. My analysis of her breast cancer journals centers on the ways in which she found agency for herself by

resisting compulsory medical practices that silenced her body and its illness. Because my book takes its title from Lorde's prose, I use her work as
a model for transforming the way we think about breast cancer. In particular, I suggest that her critique of the breast cancer establishment provides us with the most complex way of examining the intersection of the
personal—race, class, gender, sexuality—and the political—the environmental causes of the disease. Thus, my final chapter brings us full circle to
many of the issues Carson presented both in her public writing and in
her private letters.

As a whole, *Beyond Slash, Burn, and Poison* offers new insights into the
politics of breast cancer in twentieth-century U.S. literature, insights that
reflect and shape the sometimes deadly disease and its politics. Although
this book contributes to the history of breast cancer by examining the
subject through the lens of patient-centered texts, it also enables readers
to question the compulsory nature of medical care. Finally, this book is a
call to politicize cultural studies of disease by linking the literary to political struggles, particularly the struggle to determine the relationship between cancer and the environment.

CHAPTER 1

Miss Carson Goes to Washington

RACHEL CARSON'S PUBLIC SILENCE

WHEN BIOLOGIST Rachel Carson stepped into a Senate hearing in 1963 to give her testimony regarding the hazardous use of pesticides by the U.S. Department of Agriculture (USDA), Senator Abraham Ribicoff introduced her with an allusion to one of her literary ancestors: "You are the lady who started all this. . . . I think that all people in this country and around the world owe you a debt of gratitude for your writings and for your actions toward making the atmosphere and the environment safe for habitation, not only by human beings but for animals and nature itself."[1] His declaration echoed a remark made by President Abraham Lincoln in response to Harriet Beecher Stowe's novel *Uncle Tom's Cabin*; in a similar spirit Lincoln suggested that Stowe was the little white lady who wrote a book that instigated the Civil War. Other members of Congress shared Ribicoff's sense that Carson's *Silent Spring*— a book summoning the modern-day environmental movement—would change the course of history.[2] In that same hearing, Senator Ernest Gruening drew an even more explicit analogy between the two authors: "Miss Carson, every once in a while in the history of mankind a book has appeared which has substantially altered the course of history. I think that sometimes those books are in fiction form and sometimes not. One can think of many examples, such as *Uncle Tom's Cabin*, for instance. Your book is of that important character, and I feel you have rendered a tremendous service."[3]

Gruening's remarks foreshadowed the enduring impact of *Silent Spring*. But they also suggest that Carson's warnings elicited an affective and gendered public response that was akin to the empathic reactions to Stowe's novel. To be sure, Carson's narrative is not sentimental; it is an exhaustively researched scientific study written in a style that matches Henry

David Thoreau's prose more precisely than Stowe's. But it is the style of public outcry that moves Gruening to link the two texts. That particular response is gendered, raced, and classed because it posits that white, middle-class affective norms govern reactions to political crises. And indeed white, middle-class citizens felt a tremendous emotional charge from the findings in Carson's research. It is no wonder, then, that some critics felt threatened by the warnings Carson issued in her book despite the fact that her small, white frame was not the least bit intimidating; *Silent Spring* unleashed enough concern that a week-long Senate hearing was convened to explore the public health implications of insecticides.

The power of the statements by senators who listened attentively to Carson's testimony and questioned her recommendations about the toxicity of pesticides was profound. In this hearing, Carson's impeccable research stood up against the claims of the chemical corporations, whose employees testified to the safety of their products. The stakes were high: because of the tendentious arguments she made in her book, she could not risk being discredited; she did not have a wealthy corporation (as did the agricultural industry) or a prestigious university (as did most of the white, male scientists opposing and supporting her) backing her crusade. She worried about corporations looking for ways to undermine her efforts to control widespread carcinogenic pesticide use. *Silent Spring* catapulted a biologist into the limelight of Washington and the nation. Because Carson believed in her research—and knew how the government system operated after working for sixteen years, most of her adult life, for the U.S. Fish and Wildlife Service—she sacrificed her privacy, to a certain extent, for the sake of long-term public and ecological health.[4]

But one aspect of her personal life in particular would remain removed from public view: the status of her physical health. At the time of this hearing, Carson was treating her breast cancer with radiation, one of the many dangerous carcinogenic substances discussed in her book. Indeed, Carson makes this link explicitly in her chapter on cancer, which is entitled "One in Every Four": "The battle of living things against cancer began so long ago that its origin is lost in time. But it must have begun in a natural environment, in which whatever life inhabited the earth was subjected, for good or ill, to influences that had their origin in sun and storm and the ancient nature of earth" (*Silent* 219). She suggests that while radiation from the sun may be nature's way of causing cancer, "with the advent of man the situation began to change, for man, alone of all forms of life, can create cancer-producing substances, which in medical terminology are called carcinogens" (*Silent* 219). In other words, like pesticides, radiation accumulates in human and animal bodily tissues and produces known and unforeseen health problems down the line.[5] She worried that if her radiotherapy became common knowledge, that information could be used to discredit or undermine her role as a biologist and attention would be fixated on her private life instead of her public work.

Carson dealt with an array of health problems including breast cancer. She hid the most life-threatening of these illnesses for numerous reasons. Michael Warner offers one insight into Carson's desire for privacy: "In earlier varieties of the public sphere, it was important that images of the body *not* figure importantly in public discourse. The anonymity of the discourse was a way of certifying the citizen's disinterested concern for the public good" (242). In other words, Carson kept her breast cancer secret because in order to maintain the veil of scientific objectivity it was important that she remain disembodied. If *Silent Spring* convinced the public that various properties—including radiation—caused cancer, it would be risky to open up her health status to the chemical corporations' scrutiny.[6] She confided her concern to a friend: "I suppose it's a futile effort to keep one's private affairs private. Somehow I have no wish to read of my ailments in literary gossip columns. Too much comfort to the chemical companies."[7] As one who bore witness for nature, as biographer Linda Lear aptly described her, Carson needed to be perceived as an objective scientist and concerned citizen who spoke out on behalf of the public good.

Other social forces as well guided Carson's decision to keep quiet about her cancer: in the 1960s cancer itself—let alone breast cancer—was not a subject of public discussion. Nevertheless, the decision to maintain a code of secrecy about her breast cancer ensured that the public would not weep over her as some tragic figure, but if they wept at all, they would do so over concern for the state of the planet and its inhabitants more generally. The affective charge Carson carefully groomed, in fact, mobilized concerned citizens into action.

In this chapter I consider the tension between private and public as Carson straddled this line and as it set in motion prominent paradigm shifts in breast cancer research and activism that were evident by the end of the twentieth century. Perhaps for a twenty-first-century audience, used to constant disclosure of personal lives, Carson's silence about her breast cancer may appear tragic; however, the rewards of her silence were significant changes in U.S. public policy regarding the environment, which likely saved countless lives by minimizing and regulating the use of carcinogenic chemicals. Much of her story and her secrecy can be understood best in the context of the cold war, during which the only cancer that was discussed in public was Communism. This historical backdrop can be viewed most clearly in the most potent claims Carson made about cancer in *Silent Spring* and in her earlier book, *The Sea around Us,* in addition to criticism leveled against her person and her research. But most of her reflection about her struggle with her health she shared only in private letters to friends, including her doctor; layered in these documents are her primary concerns: treating her breast cancer with radiation and protecting the environment from substances like DDT (dichloro-diphenyl-trichloroethane) and atomic fallout.

Although Carson's letters about breast cancer did not have a direct effect on medical practices or breast cancer legislation, her book *Silent Spring* did. This chapter engages with the tension between her private writing and her public writing, dramatizing a historical moment before breast cancer became a public subject. Carson's scientific research continues to shape the way some scientists approach cancer research. Therefore, this chapter concludes with a look at some of the most promising changes in that research—all of which derive a method and a set of practices from *Silent Spring*.

GOING PUBLIC

In the summer of 1962, a few months prior to *Silent Spring*'s September publication date, excerpts from the book appearing in the *New Yorker* alerted the public, the government, and the chemical corporations to its provocative argument.[8] Most of the major corporations producing DDT—such as E. I. du Pont de Nemours & Co. and Velsicol Chemical Company—requested proofs from the publisher after reading the *New Yorker* installments. Velsicol even made veiled threats of a libel suit if Houghton Mifflin published the book.[9] Velsicol also targeted the National Audubon Society, which excerpted *Silent Spring* in its newsletter. A letter to Houghton Mifflin from Velsicol's lawyer, Louis McLean, indicated that perhaps Communism motivated Carson's political agenda. He claimed "in McCarthyite tones that Carson might be part of a conspiracy. There were, McLean suggested, 'sinister influences' at work. Their purpose was 'to create the false impression that all business is grasping and immoral, and to reduce the use of agricultural chemicals in this country and the countries of western Europe, so that our food will be reduced to east-curtain parity'" (Lear, *Witness*, 417).

As an unmarried woman who depended on her royalties to support family members as well as to cover the cost of medical treatment, Carson grew increasingly concerned about her financial vulnerability. The narrow way in which people in the public tried to define Carson was most obvious when she was critiqued on the basis of her marital and parental status. In fact, Carson was responsible for quite a few family members; as the sole breadwinner she cared for her mother, her nieces, and her grandnephew, whom she eventually adopted.[10] However, she had been prepared for such a reaction and had meticulously documented her research in ways that ultimately prevented anyone from acting on their legal threats.

The McCarthyite criticisms circulating about Carson, perhaps intended to silence her, also came from government officials. According to Lear, former Secretary of Agriculture Ezra Taft Benson made similar observations about Carson. In a letter to President Dwight Eisenhower he asked, "Why [would] a spinster with no children [be] concerned about genetics?' His explanation was that she was 'probably a Communist'" (Lear, *Witness*, 429). By invoking the terms *Communist* and *spinster* as if they provided some rationale for Carson's scientific work, Benson and those who echoed his claims cast a gendered and cold-war shadow on Carson. Not to be married and not to be a mother were in themselves suspicious because they undermined the national good. These claims were a veiled way of suggesting that spinsters are Communists because they do not reproduce and provide the nation with a new generation of workers and consumers. Some letters to the editor of the *New Yorker* identified what they deemed to be Carson's particularly feminine form of Communism. Readers faulted her for protecting nature at the expense of the economy as if a desire to keep the balance of nature were incompatible with corporate interests.

Whether Carson was a Communist is irrelevant. She was first and foremost a biologist at a time when a career as a scientist was not open to most women. An early childhood appreciation for literature and nature as well as an awareness of the increasing pollution in her home state of Pennsylvania guided her educational pursuits. Although her family was poor, both the Pennsylvania College for Women and later the Johns Hopkins University awarded her scholarships. Familial economic constraints exacerbated by the Depression prevented her from finishing her doctorate. But, fortunately, other professional avenues opened up for her even before she entered the master's program in zoology at Johns Hopkins. From her work at the Marine Biological Laboratory in Woods Hole, Massachusetts, for the U.S. Bureau of Fisheries grew a relationship between Carson and Elmer Higgins, the director of the government agency. He encouraged her to pursue a career as a government biologist, and his encouragement came to fruition when President Franklin Roosevelt created the U.S. Fish and Wildlife Service. There Carson's interest in conservation and talent for writing blended together. She researched and wrote many of the government documents published during her tenure there. On the side, she spent her energy on her creative-scientific writing until she could afford to devote herself to a full-time career as a writer. Carson's talent as a writer and scientist is evident in all her publications.

The technologies of the cold war—in both industry and government—worried Carson. One can see this concern in the beginning of *Silent Spring,* which contains this ecological critique of the dangers of atomic energy:

The most alarming of all man's assaults upon the environment is the contamination of air, earth, rivers, and sea with dangerous and even lethal materials. This pollution is for the most part irrecoverable; the chain of evil it initiates not only in the world that must support life but in living tissues is for the most part irreversible. In this now universal contamination of the environment, chemicals are the sinister and little-recognized partners of radiation in changing the very nature of the world—the very nature of its life. Strontium 90, released through nuclear explosions into the air, comes to earth in rain or drifts down as fallout, lodges in soil, enters into the grass or corn or wheat grown there, and in time takes up its abode in the bones of a human being, there to remain until his death. (6)

Indeed, within this allegorical "A Fable for Tomorrow," Carson paints a portrait of a world devastated by something akin to nuclear annihilation, "a spring without voices" (*Silent* 2). The ominous tone predicts extinction, which cannot be displaced on to a Communist threat; rather, Carson thrusts the responsibility onto "the people [who] had done it themselves" (3). Implicated in her claims are people who work for companies producing toxic substances. It is ironic that Velsicol imagined a sinister influence like Communism invading Carson's prose because she contends that synthetic chemicals and substances like atomic energy are the real sinister influence. Carson deftly parlays the post–World War II fear of radiation and its unknown effects on future generations into an analogy to pesticides, which similarly and invisibly enter into our environment, irrevocably altering it in the process. The cold war, like Carson's fable, exists in a universe of symbolism: "While the weapons of a hot war are guns, bombs, missiles, and the like, Cold War weapons are words, images, symbolic actions, and, on occasion, physical actions undertaken by covert means" (Medhurst et al. 19). Both of the substances Carson alludes to may have been dispersed openly, but hiding the danger of DDT and radiation from the public was decidedly covert, as Carson demonstrates in her book. Indeed, her comparison was apt; World War II inaugurated the use of DDT to eradicate bugs and the use of the atomic bomb to annihilate all sentient beings.[11] Unlike previous insect repellents, DDT eliminated insects rather than merely controlling populations, similar to the ways that atomic bombs work.

The destruction and technology of the cold war and the anxiety surrounding these developments framed Carson's developing ecological philosophy. After the Bikini atoll tests of nuclear weapons, she began to speak out against the destruction of people and nature. Carson's ecological and humanist perspective did not emphasize concerns of race and class per se; she did not focus on the ways in which people of color and poor people were often targeted in the testing of such substances. But her vision always encompassed plants, animals, and all humans as they would be affected by toxic substances. In her congressional testimony, as well as in much of the research about pesticides, the damage from atomic bombs was the yardstick with which to measure possible carcinogenic damage. The political move Velsicol made by trying to shift public discourse away from *Silent Spring* and onto its author resembles some cold-war rhetoric. Paul Boyer explains such maneuvering: "Atomic fear was

now . . . turn[ed] . . . in a new direction: not vaporization but commu-
nization was the great menace confronting mankind" (102–103). This is
precisely the scare tactic President Harry Truman used to shift the public's fear away from atomic bombs and toward the threat of Communism
when he addressed Congress in 1947 (Boyer 102–103).

Truman's rhetoric encouraged the purging of government employees and the targeting of invisible Communist citizens. And, in fact,
Carson had deliberated over this cold-war climate and its effects for at
least a decade prior to *Silent Spring*'s publication. She publicly protested
one such purging in 1953, when her former boss at the U.S. Fish and
Wildlife Service, Director Albert M. Day, was fired by the then–newly
elected Republican administration. Invoking the McCarthyite tone,
she entered into this public debate when she wrote a letter to the editor of the *Washington Post* speaking on Day's behalf: "It is one of the
great ironies of our time that, while concentrating on the defense of
our own country against enemies from without, we should be so heed-
less of those who would destroy it from within."[12] The deliberate allusion to McCarthyism in her statement underlined the hypocrisy of
those who wanted to protect Americans while simultaneously harming
people residing inside and outside the U.S. borders. However, she generally refrained from making such comments and continued to direct
her writing toward creating changes in public awareness, advocacy, and
policy. The government's crackdown on internal and external threats—
characterized by labeling people Communists—contributed to a culture of secrecy and silence. In public, political contexts, Carson rarely
seemed to buckle even when such labeling was directed at her. Her references to McCarthyism, then, served to engage the public on issues
that a cold war mind-set attempted to silence, a different kind of silent
spring.

What mattered most to Carson could not be silenced. And, in many
ways, facing breast cancer treatment and mortality brought a renewed
sense of urgency and purpose to her work. While recuperating from her
mastectomy, Carson revised her book *The Sea around Us*. In a new preface she argued more explicitly about the dangers of radioactive contamination of ocean life as a result of atomic energy. In the context of the
continuing damage caused by the Bikini atomic bomb tests, she discussed the effect that radioactive fallout has on fish and the way that

atomic particles travel up the food chain. Of particular concern also was the disposal of radioactive waste, which was left in the Pacific Ocean. Her revised preface addressed this problem: "It is only a matter of time until the contents of all such containers already deposited at sea will be free in the ocean waters, along with those yet to come as the applications of atomic science expand. To the packaged wastes so deposited there is now added the contaminated run-off from rivers that are serving as dumping grounds for atomic wastes, and the fallout from the testing of bombs, the greater part of which comes to rest on the vast surface of the sea" (xii). Carson supported these assertions by demonstrating the ways in which the radioactive elements harbored in the sea pose lethal hazards to marine and human life alike while simultaneously alluding to the suppression of this subject. At stake for Carson was the potential for spreading disease and destroying natural resources, and the fusion of these concerns illustrates some of the ways in which being a woman with cancer influenced her writing. She also clearly critiqued those who kept accurate scientific information about the hazards of radioactive fallout from the public.

Challenging limited or sequestered public discourse was an integral part of her reframing of *The Sea around Us*. In part she struggled in this book, and indeed in all her work, with a desire to make science accessible and available to the public in a historical moment when such an approach undermined one's authority and objectivity. Because the fallout from the U.S. bombs dropped on Hiroshima and Nagasaki as well as from U.S. weapons testing in the Pacific Islands landed in the ocean, Carson considered the biological and ecological impact that these materials could have on fish and wildlife in the region. Her concurrent concern over radioactive byproducts and the projected damage DDT would do to human life and natural resources was not an anomaly. World War II saw the first widespread usage of both carcinogenic properties. And other writers also linked these concerns—if only by implication—as in the August 1945 issue of *Time* magazine, which placed two stories side by side, one on the first atomic bomb explosion in New Mexico, the other a report on DDT as the new weapon in the war on insects. The common denominator was the fact that Carson believed the public should know about the dangers and have a voice in deciding whether these toxic substances should be widely used.

Going Private: A Silent Carson

Carson first discovered she had breast cancer at a time when health and disease generally were subjects for discussion only in the private domestic or medical spheres. Doctors tended to report medical prognoses to fathers or husbands; when women had no male escort, often they were left in the dark. Despite Carson's background in biology, these codes of medical secrecy prevailed, at times limiting what she knew about her physical health. While physicians filtered what Carson would know about her health, she too restricted what she shared with the public. Controlling which aspects of her health would enter the discursive arena prevented her bodily struggle from overshadowing the rational-critical debates about the dangers of pesticides (or "biocides," as she referred to them) and thereby undermining debate about the relative risks of environmental contaminants. In many ways her strategy worked. A possible cause-and-effect relationship between cancer and DDT and between cancer and radioactive fallout began to be debated by the general public. As people engaged in public discourse, the pressure to make science, industry, and government accountable to citizens who placed issues of public health on the front burner increased. These were some of the larger issues that provide a context for Carson's hiding her disease from the watchful eye of the public. They do not, however, explain precisely why the extent of her disease was hidden from her.

It worried Carson and her closest confidants that she would need to delicately balance her private life and her public role, especially after the publication of *Silent Spring*. Because she decided to keep her breast cancer secret, most of her discussions on the subject can be found in letters between Carson and her most trusted companions. Dorothy Freeman, her summer neighbor in Maine and dearest friend, received the bulk of the letters in which Carson discussed her illness as well as her intellectual projects. Concerned about her friend's mental and physical health, Freeman wrote to her about the impending significance of Carson's newest book: "Have you comprehended what the publication of *Silent Spring* is going to do to you? Once again you will be public property, no denying that."[13] In letters to Freeman Carson fleshed out her views on conservation and new technology; during "pre-*Sputnik* days, it was easy to dismiss [new technologies] as science-fiction fantasies."[14] However, Carson concedes that "the whole world of science has been revolutionized by events of the past decade or so. I suppose my thinking began to be affected soon after atomic science was firmly established."[15] In this letter, written as she was beginning to solidify the ideas that she eventually published in her landmark book, Carson creates an important link between science fiction and atomic energy. Cold-war weapons testing shifted her perspective from looking at atomic weapons as futuristic entities to fearing their realistic ability to destroy the natural world.

Strains of silence and secrecy permeate Carson's letters to Freeman on a couple of different levels. First, as can be seen above, there was a general desire to protect Carson's privacy, which both women believed could preserve her health. To that end, not disclosing personal information was essential. Second, they maintained a strict code of confidence about the nature of their relationship. Indeed, elsewhere in the above-quoted letter Freeman tells Carson, "As for the letters, darling, when I finished talking to you I decided for your peace of mind I must burn them. It seems tragic. If I start reading them I know it would be doubly hard so I think I'll just close my eyes and let them warm me for a final time."[16] The tone and tenor of this letter, like all the correspondence between these women, reveal a level of intimacy that does not have a name. Therefore dealing with Carson's letter writing itself means confronting a silence embedded in language. Because English is so limited when it comes to describing intimate relationships, to contemporary readers their friendship, as revealed in their extant letters, seems decidedly lesbian. However, neither woman used that word to define herself, and Freeman was married to a man. If pressed to characterize their relationship I would look to the nineteenth-century model of romantic friendship.[17]

Romantic friendships, one form of which is called Boston marriage, were intimate relationships between women that could also be sexual. The demonstrative language and affectionate sentiment in Freeman and Carson's letters suggest such a relationship in many respects. From the incipient stages of their correspondence in the early 1950s, this intimacy can be seen even in surviving letters. In one such note Carson reveals her feelings to Freeman: "Do you remember what someone said to the effect that (I'm quoting very inexactly) if he had two pennies he would use one to buy bread and the other to buy 'a white hyacinth for his soul'? You, dearest, are the 'white hyacinth' in which I invest part of my time—and I couldn't invest all of my time pennies in the 'bread' of the book, even for two months, if it meant giving up all that you do for me."[18] This letter, dated February 6, 1954, became a touchstone for both women. They celebrated that date annually as an anniversary, sending loving letters and hyacinth bouquets. This letter solidified the mutual devotion they felt for one another. So too did additional mailings. Because Carson was the head of her household and Freeman was married, when they wrote to one another, they did so with the understanding that the letters would be read publicly in their respective families. To ensure some level of privacy, both women began writing letters they called "apples," which they did not share with their families. These apples—reminiscent of a nineteenth-century generic form of letter writing itself—were among the destroyed letters.

Shortly before Carson's death, Freeman elaborates her fear—although without naming it—that someone might misinterpret the nature of their relationship: "So darling, please take the step NOW. I really am uneasy about [the letters]. In the *Sat. Review* I read about Dorothy Thompson's correspondence that went to Syracuse [University Library's special collections] and there was one statement that really frightened me—I don't want to put it in writing but I'll just say that the same implication could be implied about our correspondence. So, dear, please use the Strong Box quickly. We know even such volume [of our letter writing] could have its meanings to people who were looking for ideas."[19] The "strong box" is the term they used to refer to the letters marked for destruction. The anxiety expressed in this letter over journalist Dorothy Thompson alludes to the fear that their relationship could be inferred to be a lesbian one. Although some critics could easily surmise Freeman's worst fear from reading the extant letters, I think it is equally important to honor their relationship and not define it in terms they were expressly wary of. Instead, it is more productive, for my purposes, to examine the layers of privacy and secrecy that colored their bond, a bond which gave Carson a refuge from the public sphere.

I digress here to contextualize the relationship between Carson and Freeman because it speaks to the larger issues of silence and secrecy in Carson's public and private writing. Moreover, one of the two epithets hurled at Carson by critics of *Silent Spring*—*spinster*—has often had overtones that connote lesbianism. And, during Joseph McCarthy's reign, "Commie" was often used in conjunction with its derogatory male counterpart, "faggot." One common effect of all these derisive words was to induce silence in some citizens, who refused to name names. The fear of being labeled a "commie" was often enough to encourage people to implicate other possible communists. Silence, then, carries a variety of complex meanings when it comes to reviewing Carson's life. And indeed some crucial nuances need to be explored when reading her biographical documents.

A disconcerting kind of silence and secrecy emerges when one attempts to piece together her cancer history. Carson's first breast cyst appeared in 1947, although doctors diagnosed it as benign. By 1950 another one appeared, and a surgeon removed the "walnut-size" lump. To ascertain her prognosis at the time, "Rachel specifically asked . . . whether the tissue biopsy showed any evidence of malignancy, she was told it did not" (Lear, *Witness*, 185). Ten years later she discovered several other cysts in her left breast. On April 3, 1960, she admitted herself to Doctor's Hospital in Washington, D.C., where surgeon Fred R. Sanderson performed a radical mastectomy.[20] Biographer Lear notes that Carson specifically inquired about the pathology report after the surgery to determine whether her doctor had detected any signs of malignancy: "Sanderson told her she had 'a condition *bordering on malignancy*,' implying the mastectomy had been a precautionary measure. He recommended no further treatment."[21] Without any choice or voice in the matter, Carson unknowingly submitted to a Halsted radical mastectomy, the dominant surgical method at the time.

That Carson, an informed scientist, did not have any agency in deciding her surgical fate indicates the medical climate during the 1950s and 1960s in the United States. But an even more alarming fact about Carson's encounter with her physicians is that they deceived her. In a letter from Carson to her editor and friend Paul Brooks she reveals: "I know now that I was not told the truth last spring at the time of my operation. The tumor was malignant, and there was even at that time evidence that it had metastasized, for some of the lymph nodes also were found to be involved. But I was told none of this, even though I asked directly."[22] Although it is baffling that Sanderson kept his diagnosis a secret, it is equally unclear why, given his report of malignancy, he failed to recommend any further treatment.

Some of Carson's retrospective insight into the way she navigated the medical system came from her burgeoning friendship with Cleveland surgeon George "Barney" Crile, who became a pivotal figure in the fight to give women a voice in determining their surgical fate. As one of Carson's confidants he assisted her in comprehending the biology of her disease while simultaneously offering her the example of another scientist dedicated to creating an accessible prose for a popular audience at a time when such gestures constituted professional suicide. Crile and Carson shared much including the type of criticism leveled against them for trying to make science understandable to the public. With Crile's first venture into public writing, *Cancer and Common Sense,* he empowered citizens to understand treatment options and to make their own choices. Both writers encouraged their audiences to question scientific theories and practices. The relationship with Crile and his wife, Jane, was established when Carson visited Cleveland in late 1951 on a book tour promoting the first edition of *The Sea around Us.* Ten years later, after their friendship grew through their shared interest in the sea, Carson read Crile's book and was encouraged to question the sincerity of her doctors and their diagnosis.

Crile's unconventional approach to caring for patients—his own and those who read his books—provoked some of the same organizations that preferred Carson to remain silent about the environment. Because Halsted's work was so firmly codified in medical school curricula, professionals in organizations like the American Medical Association (AMA) attacked Crile, who had dared to challenge their authority. Similarly, Carson became a foe of the AMA first when she publicly critiqued its sluggish response to the health effects of pesticides on humans and later when she spoke before the Women's National Press Club. In this talk she leveled a much harsher criticism: "The AMA, through its newspaper, has just referred physicians to a pesticide trade association for information to help them answer patients' questions about the effects of pesticides on man. I am sure physicians have a need for information on this subject. But I would like to see them referred to authoritative scientific or medical literature—not to a trade association whose business it is to promote the sale of pesticides" (Carson, *Lost,* 208–209). Publicly indicting the AMA by charging that it placed financial concerns over medical concerns led to a contentious relationship between the organization and Carson. Her sense that it was more interested in a relationship with industry later carried over to her belief that it kept alternative medical remedies from the public. That Carson and Crile were both subjected to the AMA's scrutiny made it especially easy for her to trust his medical opinion.

The camaraderie between Carson and Crile grew out of a shared interest in nature and science, but it proved to be especially enlightening when her breast cancer metastasized and she sought advice from him. Questions of toxic treatment loomed large in her mind as she wondered whether to submit to standard treatment. She requested his opinion: "Which of a variety of treatments would make sense? I don't want to get into the hands of an overzealous surgeon. And I know too well that both radiation and chemo-therapy are two-edged swords."[23] In the process of helping Carson to make this decision, Crile carefully scrutinized her records, a study that unearthed the document indicating that Sanderson misled her after the initial pathology report.[24] After assessing her situation Crile concurred with her Washington medical team, recommending that she proceed with radiation treatments, and he helped her to select Ralph Caulk as her radiologist.[25]

In lengthy, elaborate letters to Dorothy Freeman, Carson details her hesitancy about those radiation treatments and the ways radiation exacerbated other ailments and produced new ones as well. While speculating about the status of the tumor as hormone dependent, Carson alleviates her friend's concerns by invoking Crile's guidance and authority,

Only one more treatment in this series. The ulcer has been painful, but today is yielding to diet and increased medicine. Dr. Caulk says it is not unusual for radiation to cause an ulcer flare up, and advised consulting Dr. Healy. I did, but knowing the routine by this time, was already doing everything necessary. Darling, we wouldn't let a little thing like a misbehaving ulcer interfere with our visit! A cold, yes—but not that. Besides, once the radiation stops, it should clear up promptly.

I continue to feel the swelling is going down. Really, this is very, very good. As I understood Dr. Crile's estimate, the chances it would do so on withdrawal of hormone stimulation were 50–50. Of course it *will* when treated directly, but the knowledge it is hormone-dependent (when confirmed) gives us additional weapons for the future. Had we continued the direct radiation in the beginning we'd never have known.[26]

Here, as in earlier letters, her optimism about the tumor shrinking eclipses her skepticism.

Crile's trusted expertise comforted Freeman and Carson. It seems they respected his wisdom even more after Carson learned that Crile's wife, Jane, had also struggled with breast cancer. She shares this story about Jane with Freeman: "Her revelation, so calmly and matter-of-factly made, somehow made my spirits soar like a shot of psychological adrenaline. . . . Now to know she, too, has encountered this shadow and in spirit at least has triumphantly overcome it is a wonderful example."[27] Carson composed her words at a time when breast cancer was not talked about in public and really not even in private. Indeed, only rarely do the words *cancer* or *breast* surface in Carson's letters—even in those discussing her medical treatment and evaluation—although Carson could be certain that Freeman understood the meaning of her euphemistic revelations. (To be sure, as Ellen Leopold points out, at this time, "breast cancer was a disease with no separate identity and no history. Until after the Second World War, cancer was considered more a monolithic disease than a vast collection of different diseases with widely different biologies and behaviors" [*A Darker* 113]. This remained the case until shortly after Carson's death.) The fact that Jane Crile shared this information with Carson is illuminating because she did so at a time when women with breast cancer did not gather together in groups or even in pairs to discuss their medical history or prognoses. And yet this camaraderie indicates why this disease was destined to become a topic of public conversation.

To shield her cancer from the public eye Carson sometimes offered explanations about her health that related to other illnesses she suffered from; one of the most debilitating of these was arthritis, which was worsened by the radiation treatments. As more medical obstacles arose and as the treatments involved more experimental applications, Carson's expertise and interest as a biologist enabled her to take a more active role. Carson's rheumatologist, Darrell Crain, consulted with Caulk to help ease the effect of radiation therapy on her arthritis. As Carson wrote to Crile, "He [Crain] might want to use intramuscular injections of gold. As you know, I'm not an especially tractable patient, and don't just go along with such things without doing some inquiring and thinking on my own. I know just enough about the use of gold to be reluctant. I know, for example, that one of its toxic effects can be exerted on the bone marrow.

My feeling about this is that I've already had to subject my bone marrow to a certain abuse via radiation."[28] She revealed her increasing misgivings to Freeman two days before her checkup with Caulk: "I am also feeling somewhat upset about this proposed treatment. Of course, I've already had a taste of having to submit to something I knew was dangerous and in theory undesirable (the radiation) but there the alternative left no choice. Here I feel I'd rather endure some arthritis than gamble with the bone marrow. Especially since it has already been under attack."[29] Carson describes the influx of toxic materials that continue to alter her body's chemistry and exacerbate other health problems in ways that are reminiscent of her writing about the effect of pesticides and radioactive fallout on the planet. As this letter conveys, Carson acquires agency in her treatment, and as a result she sees no compelling evidence of its merit. Crile investigated Crain's proposed course of treatment, and, according to Leopold, he suggested that perhaps "nitrogen mustard mixed with cortisone and injected directly into the joints" might offer better results (*A Darker* 136). Ultimately Carson decided against the gold treatment because she knew from reading pharmacological resources how incompatible her medications were:

> Besides what I've already told you, I had further and conclusive reasons for my stand. From my work at the N.I.H. [National Institutes of Health] library, I was familiar with the standard reference work on the pharmacology of various drugs, and knew that details were always included on any adverse effects, precautions to be taken, etc. . . . The whole picture of its [gold's] hazards is pretty appalling, but . . . the high point in the account is the specific and urgent statement that gold should not be administered to any person who has recently undergone a course of radiation! So there I had the answer to my own hunch. Yet, this man, knowing perfectly well I'd just had radiation, was quite ready to give it to me. What this does to my already great cynicism about doctors you can perhaps imagine.[30]

Stellar research skills, a biology background, and unyielding determination led Carson to discover an important fact that the experts to whom she entrusted her body and life had overlooked or not known. Although this time no deliberate deception kept Carson from hearing accurate information from her doctor, the episode indicates some of the hazards that can emerge when patients are not included in the decision-making process.

Carson also approached the toxic radiation with circumspection, which impelled her to investigate other treatment modalities. Leopold highlights this forward-thinking aspect when she reveals that Carson sought the advice of Morton Biskind, a nutritionist and retired toxicologist, about "nutritional approaches to her cancer, a remarkably original involvement at the time for either patient or physician" (*A Darker* 138). Carson's inquiry into these alternative treatments presented its own complexities as dietary remedies involve ingesting the chemicals contaminating the food supply: "He has great confidence in the anti-cancer factor present somewhere in the B-complex—it isn't known exactly where so that is why he urges a whole-liver preparation. This is borne out by research I'm familiar with—animal studies, I mean. Dr. B. has had patients on such a program who have simply had no recurrences, even though the cancer had metastasized at surgery. Of course one should also make a strong effort to eliminate the chlorinated hydrocarbons from one's food, because they cause loss of the B vitamins and also damage the liver. But civilization has made it so very difficult to do that!"[31]

Her curiosity about alternative medicine could not be separated from her concerns about the environment. Her desire to seek refuge in more naturopathic modalities stemmed from her belief in and love of nature. And yet the toxicity contaminating the environment that she proves in *Silent Spring* also made it difficult for her to rely on these exciting treatment possibilities. This impasse in her intellectual and medicinal research is significant because it represents the overlap between concerns raised in *Silent Spring* and those raised by her treatment. This example elucidates, perhaps, another reason for her compulsion for privacy about her illness, for claims she makes in letters about her medical treatment draw on her ecological theories.

Her interest in naturopathic remedies did not preclude her continuing with the radiation. And yet Carson increasingly divulged her deep ambivalence about allowing such toxic substances into her body. In a provocative letter to Freeman, she revealed the nature of her conundrum; the woman who was in the process of launching the modern environmental movement found herself submitting to radiation, which caused so much ecological damage in the world: "Dear, I want to explain what I meant about the radiation. I don't question whether it is the right thing. I know that 2-million-volt monster is my only ally in the major battle—but an awesome and terrible ally, for even while it is killing the cancer I know what it is doing to me. That is why it is so hard to subject myself to it each day. That's why I meant I would be happier if I knew less. But under the circumstances I have no choice but to accept the hazards of radiation."[32] In this lucid and candid description of her quandary, Carson offers insight into how trapped she feels as a person who succumbs to a treatment that she believes can be as dangerous as the disease itself. She describes the radiation equipment as a monster—a science-fiction creature even—but also as an ally in a war about which she feels deeply conflicted. But perhaps most distressing in this letter is her sense that there are no real alternatives. In sum, she had no choice.

Perhaps feeling as though she had little agency in her treatment made Carson more determined to maintain control over other aspects of her life. When she found more curiously enlarged lymph glands, her discovery indicated not only that the radiation she felt ambivalent about was not working but that, arguably, it caused a cancer recurrence. She describes this ordeal as her own "little private hell."[33] Her personal struggle began to take on even more urgency and secrecy as the publication date of *Silent Spring* in book form and in the *New Yorker* installments approached. These concerns led Carson to draft a letter to Freeman to make certain that no one would find out about her health:

> You know something of how I feel about this, but probably not the depth of that feeling. There is no reason even to say I have not been well. If you want or think you need give any negative report, say I had a bad time with iritis [inflammation of the iris] that delayed my work, but it has cleared up nicely. And that you *never saw me look better.* Please say that. If you look at my picture you will know you can say it truthfully. It is what everyone says. I know what happens when even an inkling of the other situation gets out. . . . Whispers about a private individual might not go far; about an author-in-the-news they go like wildfire. So let people think I am as well as I look.[34]

Her powerful comments to Freeman perhaps sound as though she merely wanted to avoid seeing her name in the gossip columns. Although she never explicitly states that her trepidation extended beyond this possibility, I would argue that Carson's sentiment grew out of her panic that the chemical corporations might use her ill health as a way to discredit her scientific research. Sandra Steingraber, whose work has been instrumental in expanding Carson's scientific and literary legacy, concurs on this point: "This decision [to keep breast cancer from the public] was intended to retain the appearance of scientific objectivity as she was documenting the human cost of environmental contamination. She also wished to yield her enemies in industry no further ground from which to launch their personal attacks" (*Living*, 25). As it turned out, the publicity swarming around her book (especially as second-wave feminism had yet to take center stage) indicated that she had wisely and cautiously predicted her circumstances.

In October 1962, Carson visited the Crile family in Cleveland while attending a reception and a book signing for *Silent Spring*. On this occasion, she reports to Freeman, she felt a "menacing shadow" over the public recognition she received for her writing and laborious scientific study; she does not reveal specifically what this "menacing shadow" is, but instead adds, "So many things to say, were we together!"[35] By December Carson had mixed news: she had authored a groundbreaking book that became a *New York Times* bestseller, and the cancer had metastasized in her bones. Suspecting an untraceable metastasis, Crile and Caulk concurred that more radiation treatments would offer palliative care for the pain at least and would keep the cancer from spreading at best. Moreover, Carson, likely because of the excessive and extensive radiation, began to have chest pains. After consulting with cardiologist Bernard Walsh, she informed Freeman that the heart trouble "is radiation-caused."[36] Walsh's recommended "rest cure" forced her to refrain from performing any strenuous tasks or participating in any activities, and as a result she was extremely isolated.[37] Carson's writing entered the public sphere, but, because of her metastasis and radiation-induced illnesses, her body became distanced from the fervent debate swirling around *Silent Spring*. This dichotomy of the public and the private enveloped her. She found herself involved in two parallel conflicts simultaneously: one with the chemical corporations and the mass media and the other with cancer.

Maintaining secrecy about her breast cancer clearly took its toll on her. Her private relationship with Freeman obviously sustained her in vital ways, as can be gleaned in one of their annual, amorous "hyacinth" letters: "Do you realize," Carson writes, "I have known you for a sixth of my life? Not as long or as generous a share as I could wish, but certainly a good, substantial fragment of anyone's life. And a fragment so very different from anything that preceded it, darling. Because you have brought so much happiness into my life—the joy of sharing loved and lovely things, companionship, comfort in sorrow and sickness. As I told you nine years ago, I had needed you without knowing quite what it was I needed—but when you came into my life I quickly realized something, at least, of the place you were to fill."[38] Clearly this relationship nurtured Carson as a life partner would, as indicated here in the language of marriage vows.

But the menacing specter of cancer cast a different light on even this vital relationship, as she tells Freeman a week later: "Remember, darling, it is just another of the series of battles I knew I must face, and I am sure it is not the last. We will win this one. You know the lymph tumors are very susceptible to radiation."[39] The tone here, compared with that of the previous letter, sounds more resigned. Later in this letter she shares the news that Jane Crile, her primary source of inspiration, has died. Perhaps she considered risky medicine even more at this stage because Jane Crile died one month prior to Carson's most recent metastasis in her bones. At this stage Carson deployed harsher language: as much as she persuaded herself and Freeman that the radiation would continue to help her, she knew the likelihood of the complications it could cause in her body. Carson commiserated with Crile about Jane's death, and, in so doing, she offered some insight into what it must have felt like for such a public figure to be so isolated during her life-and-death struggle: "Jane meant many things to me—a friend I loved and greatly admired and a tower of strength in my medical problems. When she wrote me after my visit with you two years ago, that she shared my problem, it was as though a great tide of courage flowed into me. If she, so vibrant, so gay, so full of the love of life, could live with the problem so fearlessly, I could at least try to do the same."[40]

Clearly Carson craved the companionship of another woman who embodied survival and who honored her need for private support. And yet despite that comforting friendship Carson could not be any more specific about her illness—even in a letter to her doctor, whose spouse

had just died of the disease—other than by referring to it as "the problem." Likewise, she avoids directly discussing death, which was itself a
taboo subject regardless of the cause. Although the words *cancer* and *death*
are not absent from her correspondence, she often employs a variety of
different terms; it is possible that some of her choices may stem from her
desire to carefully craft her prose and to be medically specific. These linguistic somersaults are not dissimilar to the cryptic ways in which Freeman and Carson discussed their friendship.

In this same letter Carson confesses that she required Crile's support
and advice but she feared writing to him after Jane's death. Clearly Jane's
death elicited thoughts about her own ominous prognosis: "Barney,
doesn't this all mean the disease has moved into a new phase and will
now move more rapidly to its conclusion? You told me last year that it
might stay in the lymph nodes for years, but that if it began going into
bone, etc., that would be a different story. . . . I still believe in the old
Churchillian determination to fight each battle as it comes, ('We will
fight on the beaches—' etc.) and I think a determination to win may
well postpone the final battle. But still a certain amount of realism is indicated, too. So I need your honest appraisal of where I stand."[41] Invoking
Winston Churchill's name in this letter indicates the sturdy façade that
Carson proposed to maintain. Just as Churchill refused to make peace
with Hitler during World War II, Carson implied that she would not call
a truce with the cancer. If his determination led to his victory in England, perhaps she could overcome the cancer in her body. In this vein
she continued radiation for palliative relief and to halt the cancer growth,
as Leopold indicates: "Caulk informed Crile that 'the areas treated have
undergone excellent involution [shrinkage].' Carson received further radiation to her left shoulder, which provided some benefit in terms of
pain relief, and to a left rib, which showed little improvement" (*A Darker*
143).[42] But this realistic description of Carson's condition seems far removed from Carson's impassioned resolve. Moreover, it reveals that her
odds fall short of survival.

Perhaps because of her growing frustration with standard radiotherapy, Carson delved deeper into research about experimental cancer therapies. Her inquiries helped her to reconceptualize the dominant
paradigms for treating cancer. Biskind sent her articles reporting on the
possibility of a controversial anticancer substance known as Krebiozen.

Although the articles—including one from a medical journal—did not claim that Krebiozen cured cancer, they intrigued her. She described the drug's appeal and its potential in a letter to Freeman:

> It has been a subject of bitter controversy for more than a decade, though for reasons that reflect chiefly the bickerings, struggle for power, bigotry, etc., within the medical profession rather than any valid objection to the drug. "Drug" really is a misnomer; it is an anti-cancer substance produced by living tissues (by injecting a mold preparation into horses, then extracting this substance from the blood serum). So, instead of attacking the local manifestations of the disease, as by radiation, it really helps the whole body resist. There is no claim it is 100% effective, but about 50 percent show great improvement for considerable periods, relief from pain, return to active lives, etc. A recent article in the Journal of the AMA makes a comparison of breast cancer patients treated with Krebiozen, androgens, estrogens, removal of adrenals, pituitary, etc., and the Krebiozen patients survived longer than any other. . . . It is non-toxic and it is claimed there are no side effects.[43]

Carson's comprehension of the way Krebiozen behaves made sense to her conceptually—rather than operating like a weapon that merely attacks the cancer locally, Krebiozen enables the body to become stronger so it can resist the disease systemically. Carson also found comfort in the fact that the AMA opposed the drug. The AMA was one of the organizations that fought her call for pesticide regulation and public-policy reform with respect to the consumption and production of DDT. Therefore, the AMA's position on the drug meant relatively little to her. Witnessing his patient's exhaustion from the radiation, Healy agreed to give Carson the injections of Krebiozen, although Caulk opposed her new treatment modality. Political rather than scientific differences guided Caulk's dissension from her medical choice; he worried that if it appeared to work on a public figure, the drug would garner widespread interest (Lear, *Witness,* 446).[44] From the perspective of medical professionals, "alternative" medicine detracts from the lucrative and institutionalized treatments that standard medicine provides. However, such fears made little sense in this case because the public was not aware of Carson's illness or her treatment at the time.

Eventually, Carson shared her desire to try Krebiozen with Crile. She began by offering to subject herself to further radiation if necessary despite the fact that her "poor vertebra has been bombarded" with so much radiation that she had lost track of how much her body had endured.[45] Crile supported her choice to experiment with a method that dealt with the disease systemically rather than locally. He likely wanted to support her agency in the process—despite his reservations about Krebiozen—because he also saw a correlation between her breast cancer and the environment: "Remember that the endocrine approach to the problem of breast cancer employs alterations in the specific chemicals that control the growth of specific tumors. This is the type of biological specificity that you are looking for in your ecological problems and that to date have shown the greatest promise in control of malignant tumors."[46] Crile's analogy was apt: he drew a lucid parallel between the attempt to control nature with pesticides and the attempt to conquer cancer with drugs, and he pointed to the greater efficacy of systemic approaches to controlling both cancer and the environment.

In theory Krebiozen sounded like a rational approach. In practice Leopold contends that it "had no effect on her symptoms or pain whatsoever" (*A Darker* 147). When it did not offer her the results she had hoped for, she found herself facing the radiology team once again. On returning home from the hospital, Carson promptly told Freeman: "I've been X-rayed practically from chin to ankles!"[47] And yet the cancer continued to grow, and the pain increased. After conferring with one another, Caulk and Crile decided to give her "testosterone phosphorous to ease her pain" and to enable her to walk, although ultimately this treatment too failed to offer any relief (Leopold, *A Darker,* 147). The most discouraging sign of debilitation, however, was the continued pain in her hand and arms, which made writing particularly difficult for her. It is not clear when this pain first began, and physicians could not determine whether it resulted from a metastasis. Crile thought it was related to arthritis. However, Caulk continued to order radiation to attack what he maintained could only be a metastasis.

In January Carson wrote to Freeman in an uncharacteristically matter-of-fact tone about her seriously declining health. She reported that her visit with Caulk left her intuiting "that he left unsaid, 'Don't expect too much more time.'"[48] For the first four months of 1964 her health deteriorated rapidly both from cancer metastasis and from the effects of ra-diation, which contributed to her loss of smell and taste, staphylococcal meningitis, shingles, severe anemia, and a worsened heart condition. In one last-ditch effort to fight the cancer Crile and Caulk sent her to the Cleveland Clinic for a hypophysectomy. This procedure entails "doctors implant[ing] radioactive yttrium-90 to kill functioning pituitary tissue" (Leopold, *A Darker*, 148). After poring over medical records, Lear sug-gests that Carson's "preoperative physical revealed that the cancer had metastasized into her liver. One physician noted that her heart condition made any surgery risky" (*Witness* 479). The procedure nearly killed Car-son. Eventually she stabilized enough to return to her Maryland home. She died the following month, on April 14, 1964, of a heart attack.

CARSON'S PRECAUTIONARY PRINCIPLES

That Carson died of a heart attack, a death linked to prolonged exposure to radiation, is telling.[49] The unleashing of carcinogenic sub-stances into her body—particularly at a time when doses were unregu-lated—parallels the unleashing of unregulated pesticides and radiation into the environment. During the two years before her death, she spent her time writing and speaking publicly about the hazards of poisoning the world. In one such speech, to the Kaiser Foundation Hospitals and Permanente Medical Group in San Francisco, she made these concerns explicit: "One of the most troublesome of modern pollution problems is the disposal of radioactive wastes at sea. By its very vastness and seeming remoteness the sea has attracted the attention of those faced with the problem of disposing the by-products of atomic fission. And so the ocean has become a natural burying-place for contaminated rubbish and for other low-level wastes of the atomic age. Studies to determine the limits of safety in this procedure for the most part have come after rather than before the fact, and disposal activities have far outrun our precise knowl-edge as to the fate of these waste products" (Carson, *Lost*, 235–236).

Before Carson's death, her work was vindicated, in an unfortunate incident, when five million dead fish were discovered floating belly up in the Mississippi River; the disaster caused problems for the power plants and drinking water in nearby Louisiana communities. The U.S. Public Health Service found that the fish died from trace levels of the pesticide endrin in their bodies. One year later Carson learned that "the source of the endrin in the Mississippi was a Memphis waste-treatment plant owned by none other than the Velsicol Chemical Company, the pesticide's developers" (Lear, *Witness,* 470). This public fiasco turned out to be precisely the evidence Senator Ribicoff and Secretary of the Interior Stewart Udall needed to garner congressional support for the first U.S. clean water legislation. *Silent Spring* eventually paved the way for the introduction of bills regulating pesticide in over forty state legislatures.[50]

These results succinctly reveal the impact of one New England woman who wrote with an eye toward the power narratives have to alter public policy. They also indicate the state of Carson's mind when she hid her breast cancer from the public. She did not base her decision on shameful feelings about her postmastectomy body or denial regarding the rapid metastasis of her cancer. Concealing breast cancer was, for her, not about maintaining hegemonic sex roles by feeling confined to a private, domestic sphere. Rather, Carson self-imposed this secret because she wanted to minimize the intensity of the chemical corporations' personal attacks, which emphasized her gender and her popular writing style as a way to discredit her scientific objectivity. Instead she focused on her expertise as a former employee of the U.S. Fish and Wildlife Service; this strategy enabled her to navigate the waters of secrecy and denial advanced by the government. With *Silent Spring*, she effectively fought to keep the USDA from controlling nature. Her example demonstrates the tension between private battles and public debates. Carson's ability to start a national conversation about insecticides and the environment ultimately led to changes in public policy. Ironically, her silence about her concurrent struggle with breast cancer illustrates the complexities of being public about a private illness.

While keeping her breast cancer intensely private, Carson pushed herself to make public appearances on television after the publication of *Silent Spring,* partially to squelch the rumors of her illness. However, most significant was her presence at Senate hearings when she testified as a biologist and as a citizen about the harmful use of pesticides: "Carson had been thinking about her recommendations for policy change since beginning her research five years before. . . . Rachel wanted her testimony to provide specific recommendations that would bring improvement but at the same time be politically feasible. Rather than advocate wholesale reforms, Carson's years of experience in government kept her pragmatic and made it that much more impossible for legislators to dismiss her" (Lear, *Witness*, 453). Ultimately she argued for action on the part of industry and government. Her theory, which later became known as the "precautionary principle," suggests that chemical harm can be prevented if suspicious toxins are studied before they are put on the market. In other words, the precautionary principle forces corporate and government entities to take responsibility. Carson was extraordinarily forward thinking in requesting that the government and corporations not assume that products are safe until they prove otherwise. Rather, she believed that they must determine the toxicity of any given substance before introducing it to the public in a widespread fashion.

One of the many publications honoring Rachel Carson's legacy, *Rachel's Environment & Health Weekly*, reported in 1995 that "twenty-seven peer-reviewed scientific papers and technical reports have now identified radiation as a cause of breast cancer in women. The first such report appeared in 1965"—one year after Carson's death (Montague 3). Although the findings of these studies leave little doubt as to the harmful effects of radiation, it is still advocated for diagnosis and therapy; however, the primary difference today is that most radiation doses are regulated and monitored. And this is one of the legacies Carson gave us that her critics have often overlooked or ignored: she advocated for regulating, not eliminating, the use of hazardous substances like DDT and radiation.

One of the most pressing objectives for Senator Ribicoff and his colleagues during their week-long investigation of the dangers of pesticides was contrasting the contamination and environmental harm caused by radiation and by pesticides. When he questioned Jerome Wiesner, chairman of President John F. Kennedy's Science Advisory Committee, Ribicoff wanted to know whether Wiesner could "offer some comparison between the hazards of fallout from nuclear testing and the hazards from chemical poisoning of the environments."[51] In 1963 this question was still not widely understood; and scientists and citizens could not come to any consensus on it because cold-war concerns dictated that government and industry demand secrecy about radiation. Wiesner responded by differentiating the quantity of substances used and the residue left behind: "The major difficulty that we had in trying to assess the effect of fallout was that we were dealing with very low levels of radioactivity in the environment."[52] From a historical vantage point, it is significant that radioactive fallout thus became the yardstick with which to measure all other public health and environmental concerns.

Carson knew that the public feared radioactive fallout in spite of the Atomic Energy Commission's publicity campaign promoting its safety. She recognized the potential of radiation fear to engage citizens and politicians in a crucial debate, and because pesticides and radiation could both cause cancer, she realized she could use the analogy to make the case for pesticide control. Therefore, she opened her congressional testimony with that allusion: "Contamination of various kinds has now invaded all of the physical environment that supports us—water, soil, air, and vegetation. It has even penetrated that internal environment within the bodies of animals and of men. It comes from many sources: radioactive wastes from reactors, laboratories, and hospitals; fallout from nuclear explosions; domestic wastes from cities and towns; chemical wastes from factories; detergents from homes and industries."[53] Her warning in this testimony reads like a prophecy similar to the fable that opens *Silent Spring*. Cancer maps of the United States clearly indicate that incidence and mortality rates remain far higher in communities located near polluting organizations and institutions—communities that are, not incidentally, usually made up of working-class people and people of color—than in communities that are not in polluted areas. In her statement to the Senate, she elaborated her comparison of pesticides and radioactive fallout by demonstrating that these chemicals are not static; instead, they travel in animals, water, soil, and air.[54]

During a second congressional hearing on pesticide control, Carson declared, "There is no predictable safe level of application once poison has entered the food chains."[55] In this Senate hearing she testified in support of two legislative bills that encouraged—although they did not require—a consultation with the U.S. Fish and Wildlife Service prior to any federally sponsored pesticide spraying. Questioning Carson after she read her prepared statement, Senator A. S. Mike Monroney wondered whether the pending bill suggested that "we are going to perhaps do to ourselves, in poisoning wildlife and fishery products, almost as much damage as we would do through the fallout of radioactive materials from testing."[56] Carson responded by indicating that the interrelationship of species requires concern: "We have all of these fishes in sport fishing areas, and commercial fishing areas too for that matter, that are near the end of their food chains, and they are carrying heavy residues. Many of them are going to serve as food for human beings."[57] Presenting this perspective in such a public arena allowed Carson to mobilize a concerned citizenry to support pesticide regulations. It was an important first step toward the study and analysis of public health hazards stemming from environmental pollutants.

Carson's effect on the modern environmental movement still lingers. The majority of environmental organizations honor her memory by invoking her name—the Silent Spring Institute, *Rachel's Environment & Health Weekly*, the Rachel Carson Council—as well as her beliefs and her practices. On the thirtieth anniversary of the publication of *Silent Spring*, Congress held a commemorative hearing to assess the level of pesticide use in the United States. However, the primary function of the hearing was to discuss registering chemicals, rather than to examine the carcinogenic properties of those pesticides or their toxicity levels. Moreover, despite the intention to honor Carson's memory with this hearing, no citizens were included to testify or to question the policies of the Environmental Protection Agency or the practices of the USDA.[58] The lack of citizen testimony demonstrates that the hearing was a symbolic gesture as opposed to an authentic expression of Carson's legacy. That her scientific work and activist spirit continue to motivate progressive environmentalists and politicians ultimately reveals the power of her legacy.

Of all the work that emerged from Carson's scientific writing the Silent Spring Institute, located in Cape Cod and formed in 1993, is the organization that embodies her humanist and ecological vision most precisely. At its core are the principles that Carson adhered to most devoutly in her work as a scientist and a citizen: "Silent Spring Institute is a unique partnership of scientists, physicians, public health advocates, and community activists united around the common goal of studying associations between the environment and women's health, especially breast cancer. The Institute is committed to breast cancer prevention, a research agenda with an activist vision that goes far beyond science-as-usual. To this end, we foster a different approach by crossing scientific disciplines and involving the public. This open process stimulates creative thinking while keeping our work grounded in the research questions that are critical to the women of Cape Cod" (Silent Spring Institute 2). The focus on breast cancer connects various facets of Carson's public and private writing by unveiling all the facts she could not reveal thirty years earlier.

The scientific work under way on Cape Cod and in Newton, an upper-middle-class, predominantly white, suburb of Boston, is founded uniquely on a collaborative process that works with a broad cross-section of the public. Few other scientific think tanks have an integral grassroots foundation. The scientists participate in multidisciplinary research that responds to the needs of the community and lets the public set the agenda for their research. Rather than mystifying epidemiological cancer research, these scientists work diligently to make their science accessible and to be accountable to the public. The Silent Spring Institute represents the best of what can happen when citizens enter the public sphere and set the terms of the debate, whether it be in the realm of policy or of science.[59] Using new methods of scientific research these scientists and citizens not only study current practices but also use historical data to account for changes in incidence rates and environmental pollution over time.[60]

I end with this brief gloss of the Silent Spring Institute's activities because I think it should serve as a prototype for merging future research and activism. The Silent Spring Institute's proactive approach to research has the potential to uncover the root causes of disease and to discover real ways of preventing breast cancer. When activists, scientists, and policymakers gather together rather than working separately there is a greater potential for creative approaches to scientific inquiry. For instance, in Racine, Wisconsin, in 1998, the Wingspread Conference on the Precautionary Principle avowed, "When an activity raises threats of harm to human health or the environment, precautionary measures should be taken even if some cause and effect relationships are not fully established scientifically. In this context the proponent of an activity, rather than the public, should bear the burden of proof" (Raffensperger).[61] This statement, otherwise known as the precautionary principle, asks that chemical corporations and government entities test products before exposing them to the public. Instead of asking people who are sick with illnesses like cancer to testify before Congress and actively work to hold industry and the military accountable for their harm, the precautionary principle makes the corporate entity take responsibility. This principle is precisely the motivating paradigm behind the Silent

Spring Institute, which joins forces with other environmental groups to educate the public about the need for institutionalizing this principle as a practice.

This formal statement about the precautionary principle and the work of the Silent Spring Institute are just two examples of ways that Carson's private struggle with breast cancer and her public fight to regulate toxic chemicals permeate cancer research and knowledge today. These collaborative ventures demonstrate the potential of women who are not silenced about their disease. In this respect, these scientists and citizens bear witness both to Carson's silences and to her public testimonies. In the pre–second-wave feminist era of the early 1960s there were neither models nor support for being public about one's disease. First Lady Betty Ford would intuitively change the landscape of public debates about previously private subjects, as the next chapter illustrates.

CHAPTER 2

Media Medical Interventions

BETTY FORD'S PUBLIC(ITY) PEDAGOGY

IF THE POLITICAL and cultural climate in which Rachel
Carson lived made her cautious about revealing aspects of her private life
in public, one decade after her death the tide began to turn. In the years
between Carson's death in 1964 and First Lady Betty Ford's discovery of
a breast lump in 1974, occasional first-person narratives about breast
cancer in mainstream magazines like *Ladies' Home Journal* gave way to
more frequent articles by patients and by physicians.[1] With the rise of
second-wave feminism, concerns about women's bodies captured the attention of the public in new ways; however, many of the objectives of the
women's liberation movement—and the women's health movement—
focused on young women's bodies and on white, middle-class women's
bodies.[2] As breast cancer became a topic of conversation, at least among
women in private groups or in women's magazines, it also seeped into
public discourse.

Conversation in various public and counterpublic spheres about
breast cancer slowly evolved as a result, in part, of Carson's iconoclastic
friend and medical advisor, George Crile. Over the course of twenty years
he published a wide variety of articles in medical journals challenging the
widespread use of the Halsted radical mastectomy. But with the publication of *What Women Should Know about the Breast Cancer Controversy*,
which was excerpted in the then-new feminist publication *Ms.* only a
year before Ford's diagnosis, the media and the public began to discuss
breast cancer directly. Crile, who was a refuge for Carson during her silent
struggle, circulated his ideas to help other women navigate a medical system that focused more on profit than on patients' care. Much of his motivation for writing for lay readers came from his sincere empathy for his
patients, friends, and most notably his deceased wife, Jane Halle Crile.[3]

His compassionate style of administering medicine inspired his patient Babette Rosamond to write, under the pseudonym Rosamond Campion, one of the first breast cancer memoirs. *The Invisible Worm*, published in 1972, presented a complex view of the language surrounding breast cancer prior to Ford's public announcement two years later. Although Campion wrote her book about the process of navigating the course of her own surgery in the language of choice, she did so anonymously; thus she perpetuated the legacy of breast cancer as a silent subject even in the context of a renewed feminist project regarding women's right to choose how to treat their own bodies.[4] Crile claimed that Campion's writing helped him disseminate his message (Crile, *What Women*, 13). And indeed it did. However, as Betty Ford's story reveals, Crile and Campion may have raised awareness in the public, but they did not do so in the dominant medical arena; therefore, the first lady's surgeon never advised her that she could choose to have a less mutilating surgery. This is the context for Ford's announcement about her breast cancer.

Recalling her rationale for disclosing her breast cancer diagnosis, Ford situated her health crisis in relation to President Richard Nixon's then-recent resignation. Ford went public with her illness to alter the perception of covert scandal in the White House. Accordingly, she framed her plight in the context of her husband's pardoning Nixon: "Eighteen days after the Nixon pardon, my doctors discovered that I had cancer" (197). Indeed, President Ford kept his promise to end secrecy in matters political and private.[5] In September 1974 the White House allowed Betty Ford to arrive at Bethesda Naval Medical Center before the president announced on the evening news that she would undergo a biopsy and possibly a mastectomy. Although the president made the initial public revelation about his wife's biopsy and impending Halsted radical mastectomy, they decided upon the content of the announcement together.[6] Ford's candor about her breast cancer and the mass media's engagement with this subject exposed women's lack of agency in their medical treatment and the outmoded surgical practices that Carson's experience with cancer illuminates.

By the time she learned about her disease, the subject of cancer mortality, research, and funding had seeped into the consciousness of Americans, in part because of Crile's work and in part because of Nixon's publicity campaign to advance medicine in the "war on cancer";

increased funding for the National Cancer Institute (NCI) paved the way for new surgeries, chemotherapies, radiotherapies, and comprehensive cancer centers. Popular newspapers and magazines circulated stories of survivors and of celebrity bouts with cancer. However, not until Ford and Vice President Nelson Rockefeller's wife, Happy, discovered lumps in their breasts nineteen days apart did the words *breast cancer* explode into the public consciousness through the mainstream media in a sustained fashion.

Ford's and Rockefeller's confessional rhetoric touched the public because of the honest display of emotion by the country's most public wives. Ford acquired some agency through her revelation and the ensuing media publicity, but it had its limitations. This chapter provides an analytical and historical framework for examining the role she played in creating awareness about breast cancer in the public sphere. Having the words *breast cancer* appear in the mass media ended a silence about the corporeal reality not only of the dominant surgery, the Halsted radical mastectomy, but also of the one-step biopsy-surgery process, which limited treatment options for women. To raise women's consciousness, Ford balanced her feminist values with a traditionally gendered speaking style that alleviated shame about a previously private topic and simultaneously provided a forum for discussing medical practices.

As a high-profile public figure, Ford provides us with an interesting opportunity to examine the way celebrity and publicity combine to raise awareness about an issue. On the one hand, she carefully used her position to end the silence surrounding breast cancer. On the other hand, her race and class subjectivity inadvertently ensconced the public mythology of breast cancer as a disease of affluent, white women. By analyzing Ford's writing about her illness and the publicity of it, I uncover the complex dynamic between her increased agency and the way the media undermined her public narrative. The mass media certainly helped to educate the public about the disease and its obsolete treatment; but in the process the magazines and newspapers (and of course television) represented Ford's postmastectomy body in ways that rendered it hypervisible. By tracing this historical moment, I demonstrate the ways in which the media simultaneously provided women with a newfound sense of agency and with a limited means for relaying the nuances necessary to persuade women to care for their bodies.

THE CONFESSIONAL IS POLITICAL:
WHITE-GLOVE RHETORIC

In contradistinction to Carson's silences about her illness and her relationship with Dorothy Freeman, Ford explicitly framed her narrative about breast cancer by calling attention to her role as a wife. Consequently, her autobiography falls within the generic convention of a love story. Designing the narrative as a romantic one enabled her to reel in readers with promises of tell-all tales. By insisting that her book feature stories about courtship and marriage, she secured an audience of primarily like-minded, white, heterosexual, middle-class, Republican ladies.[7] To satisfy this particular readership she denied writing a narrative about manners, yet she placed those concerns in the forefront throughout the text. For instance, she describes her concern about knowing when to wear her white gloves and when to take them off: "In Washington people in government service live pretty strictly by protocol. As a bride, I bought my first book on whether to wear gloves to a tea, and whether you take off one glove when going through a receiving line (you have to take off both gloves; you should never have just one glove on), and while these things seem silly sometimes, they make your life easier. You know what's expected of you" (72).[8]

Remarkably Ford's preoccupation with etiquette rests comfortably beside her candor about feminist issues. Wearing white gloves—coded by her race, class, and sexuality—figures prominently in the construction of herself. Wearing suitable attire and serving appropriate meals mattered to a politician's wife, but those concerns never overwhelmed her opinions (which were in fact quite progressive) about women's bodies and women's lives. In this calculated way Ford disseminated her opinions. She did not want to lose readers who equated "political" women with feminism; but she also refused to be malleable or pliant when expressing her admittedly feminist views. Moreover, she associated the term *political* with Watergate, and the president and first lady distanced themselves from the secretive discourse that plagued Nixon. Her style of speaking and writing—which I call white-glove rhetoric—at times seems duplicitous, but it is the method she relied on to shape public debates in the mass media.

In September 1974 breast cancer was still synonymous with death. With that in mind, Ford concentrated her energy on alleviating any possibility of recurrence. She understood recovery from breast cancer as "a question of mental health affecting your physical health" (203), and she survived by dealing with the particularly difficult psychological effects of losing her right breast. As a part of her healing process she imagined how she would have reacted if her husband had had a body part amputated: "If he'd lost a leg, I wouldn't have deserted him, and I knew he wouldn't desert me because I was unfortunate enough to have had a mastectomy. Neither of us could walk away from the other. When I say we've had an ideal marriage, I'm not just talking about physical attraction, which I imagine can wear pretty thin if it's all a couple has built on. We've had that and a whole lot more" (206). Clearly, this is a description of an emotionally sustaining marriage. Yet Ford's comparison of her breast to her husband's leg is rather shocking.[9] Because losing a breast called attention to her sexual body, Ford deflected that attention by juxtaposing it and an imagined loss of her husband's leg. Such an image resonated profoundly with a public witnessing so many wounded Vietnam veterans returning without their limbs. Moreover, nowhere in this passage does Ford name her lost body part. The absence of the word *breast* indicates some of her cunning style. By comparing a breast to a leg, she desexualized herself by downplaying the breast's sexual and gendered connotations. At the same time Ford makes breast cancer intelligible precisely because she presents herself as relatively chaste. At fifty-six she had already borne her children, and, therefore, she was not potentially a nursing mother. This presentation of herself as rather monastic kept the story from spiraling into a voyeuristic tale—as it might have if Jacqueline Kennedy had been the subject.[10]

Ironically, Ford reassured readers that her marriage remained physical at the same time that she undermined that aspect of it. She seems oblivious to the social and cultural significance of her breast.[11] But breasts—most often youthful, white breasts—are different than legs because they are sexual and they are fetishized. Zillah Eisenstein makes the sexual and racial aspects of female breasts clear: "The breast, in representing femininity, is simultaneously implicated in whiteness. The female body, despite its racial identity and multiplicity of colors, exists as a fantasized icon. The fantasy parades despite the many ways that reality negates it. Variety is displaced by singularity; color becomes white. And, the white body becomes a universalized abstraction: thin, large breasted,

small waisted, with blonde hair" (141). Ford had little control over the
way the media portrayed her illness. And in this sense she likely had no
awareness of the ways in which her identity as a white, privileged woman
reiterated the belief that breast cancer affects only older, middle-class,
white women. The danger in unconsciously circulating these myths
about race and cancer can be gleaned from the collected statistics of
women who visited NCI and ACS centers as a result of Ford's public disclosure. Data from the NCI and ACS Breast Cancer Detection Demonstration Project (BCDDP) indicated that "the majority of the BCDDP
participants were white (88.3 percent). Only a small percentage of the
population was black (5.3 percent) or Oriental (3.0 percent)" (Baker
196, 202). Thus, we can conclude that women who visited the centers
tended to be white.

In some respects it was not only Ford's body that visibly marked her
race in this context but also the discursive choices she made. Using
a confessional style for speaking and writing, Ford plugged into the
consciousness-raising discourse of mainstream, white feminism. Rita Felski links confession and consciousness raising by resuscitating both terms
in ways that highlight the political potential of both: "Like consciousness-raising, the confessional text makes public that which has been private, typically claiming to avoid filtering mechanisms of objectivity and
detachment in its pursuit of the truth of subjective experience" (87–88).
Confession afforded Ford an appropriate speaking style for a first lady,
but it simultaneously relegated her to the realm of women's consciousness raising. This model accommodated her history of being quite candid
in public. In her autobiography she characterizes her story as romantic
and therefore not political; however, her life took a marked turn toward
the public and the political when she received fifty thousand letters from
cancer survivors after her mastectomy.

But Ford had already established this pattern of carefully balancing
secrecy and speaking out in public about her personal struggles. About a
nervous breakdown she experienced in 1965, the result of pressures of
being a politician's wife, she confided: "I don't believe in spilling your
guts all over the place, but I no longer believe in suffering in silence over
something that's really bothering you. I think you have to get it out and
on the table and discuss it no matter what it is" (137). Ford developed
this philosophy during her psychiatric treatment, which demystified

prevalent stereotypes of women and madness for her. Sharing these experiences alleviated some of the shame Ford felt about her nervous breakdown.[12] For instance, as first lady, she spoke at a national meeting of psychiatrists and later said of this speech: "I'd had psychiatric care, and . . . I thought it was just as important to take care of your mind as it was to take care of your body. I got a standing ovation. Because so many people think it's shameful to confess that they can't make it alone, that it's an admission of something terribly wrong with them. There was nothing terribly wrong with me" (139).

In moments like this Ford realized the persuasive power of confession. Her statement represents a shift between polite, white-glove rhetoric and the politically astute rhetoric of the president's wife. When she revealed her experiences, taboo topics like mental illness, usually reserved for private discussion, became public as she erased some of the stigma attached to them. Ford's pattern for effecting change retrospectively—and at times self-consciously—through her personal experiences derived much of its power and context from the second-wave feminist dictum that the personal is political.[13]

Ford insisted on publicly discussing subjects most often regarded as private. When Barbara Walters interviewed her, for instance, Ford prefaced her remarks by stating that she "didn't want to talk about anything political." Walters responds to this criterion rather cannily by posing one of the most political questions she could ask: she seeks Ford's opinion of the Supreme Court's then-recent ruling on abortion. Without hesitation Ford replies: "I said I agreed with the Supreme Court's ruling, that it was time to bring abortion out of the backwoods and put it in the hospitals where it belonged" (167). In her autobiography, Ford did not analyze the contradictory nature of her previously articulated boundaries and her comment on a political subject except to say that with her statement on abortion "my reputation for candor was established" (167). Here is Ford at her paradoxical best, insisting on having no political agenda while unveiling one. She constructs a distinction between private and political, but she repeatedly collapses it. This interview suggests a significant parallel between a woman's right to choose with respect to reproduction and with respect to breast cancer. Ford's performance makes it clear that nonpolitical ladies can support a woman's right to control her body. Ford cultivated a strategy in which she personalized her experiences to make herself appear less threatening to a mass audience. Confession allowed her to initiate public debates that could lead to political change by walking a fine line between the lady in the white gloves and the radical women's liberationist in the streets.[14]

This pattern enabled Ford to relieve the stigma of breast cancer and shape public debates. Jürgen Habermas's analysis of the bourgeois public sphere explains why Ford's rhetoric reached a mass public audience and why the media spectacle ensued. In Habermas's explication of the bourgeois public sphere, private citizens are constituted as a public through their discourse. He contends that public discourse can form the basis of democracy. Public debates in the media, for instance, help set the issues that legislators ultimately decide on. When the system works at its best, those with power do not determine what gets discussed in the public sphere. From Habermas's perspective, however, personal experience as conveyed in a confession would not be an effective mode of discourse because it is subjective. But, in fact, women, people of color, and poor people, who often use subjective, personal experiences to create public debates, have not been entirely absent from the public sphere, as Nancy Fraser articulates: "The view that women were excluded from the public sphere turns out to be ideological; it rests on a class- and gender-biased notion of publicity, one that accepts at face value the bourgeois public's claim to be the public. In fact, . . . the bourgeois public was never the public" ("Rethinking" 7).

I would argue that because Ford's white-glove rhetoric captured the dominant public's attention she functioned as an effective carrier of public opinion to a wide variety of citizens. To be sure, in the 1970s few in the dominant public indicated that they wanted to hear about breast cancer. Much to the astonishment of publishers, politicians, and physicians, after the revelation of Ford's illness, breast cancer clearly captured public interest. In her interviews and in her autobiography she addressed an audience to some extent like herself—white, middle-class, heterosexual ladies—the majority of whom were not living as political wives in Washington, D.C. Because Ford laced her white-glove rhetoric with the views of a Gloria Steinem feminist who believed everything is political, she sometimes seemed like a paradoxical figure.[15] By making her autobiography a heterosexual love story, for example, she seemingly disavowed the powerful political lessons of her text—but she accessed an audience that overt feminists like Steinem could not always reach.

The sometimes politically shrewd manner in which Ford negotiated her way can best be understood by examining a passage of her autobiography: "The one thing that worried me was whether I'd be able to wear my evening clothes again. Jerry said I was silly. 'If you can't wear 'em cut low in front, wear 'em cut low in back'" (210). In this dialogue the first lady confesses a common fear among women with breast cancer. Because she wrote this passage in retrospect, she knew of her initial effect on other breast cancer survivors. Thus, when she expresses her anxiety about life in a postmastectomy body she recognizes the power it holds for her readers. She compares her experiences to those of women who wrote to her with their stories about their scarred bodies. Other women declared timidity when it came to looking at themselves in the mirror. Ford's curiosity about her scar led her to sneak peeks beneath her bandage. Yet the very nature of her celebrity increased her angst—not about her body in intimate settings with her husband as readers might expect, but about people glaring at her in public. Her apprehension about dressing her body for the public stems from her heightened awareness that others would constantly gaze at her body trying to recall which breast she lost (likely because she wore a prosthesis). Having to display her body as a part of her role as first lady obliged her to struggle with her wound; unlike the women who corresponded with her, she had to endure the harsh lens of the media and the public's response.

PUBLIC PEDAGOGY:
TEACHING BREAST CANCER 101

To say that Ford's candor about her breast cancer granted a unique pedagogical opportunity to the mass media is an understatement. No one was more aware of this didactic potential than Ford, as she explains in her autobiography: "I got a lot of credit for having gone public with my mastectomy, but if I hadn't been the wife of the President of the United States, the press would not have come racing after my story, so in a way it was fate. . . . Even before I was able to get up, I lay in bed and watched television and saw on the news shows lines of women queued up to go in for breast examinations because of what happened to me"

(203). Her narrative clarifies her comprehension of the immense and immediate impact of her disclosure. And yet by characterizing her opportunity to educate the public as fate, she denies her agency on some level. Her previous experiences speaking out on subjects like abortion did not prepare her for the impact of the breast cancer publicity. She now realizes that her straight talking, as she defines it, could raise the consciousness of others:

> Lying in the hospital, thinking of all those women going for cancer checkups because of me, I'd come to recognize more clearly the power of the woman in the White House. Not *my* power, but the power of the position, a power which could be used to help. I felt I hadn't even begun to work effectively for the causes—the Equal Rights Amendment, mental health, the fight against child abuse, the fight against the abuse of old people and retarded people—that I cared about. Even so, I'd been given all kinds of credit for such straight talking as I'd already done. Betty Friedan told reporters I'd been so good for the women's movement she hoped "some of our strength can flow back to her." (212)

Even though she identifies a source of agential power here, she distinguishes it from herself—that is, she sees her ability to be a public pedagogue as related to her role and not to her voice. The revelation Ford describes can be defined as a "click!" experience—a moment when she shifts her consciousness and she connects her actions and thoughts to the larger framework of feminism. Lisa Hogeland places the spread of consciousness raising in the 1970s in the context of women's responses to similar gestures: "Like the personal essays that were a staple of feminist periodicals in the 1970s—the 'click!' letters to *Ms.,* for example, in which women described some small experience that crystallized their understandings of women's oppression," consciousness-raising groups provided a forum that connected women and often propelled them into action (24). For the first lady, this experience contributed to the development of her voice; it created a more conscious corporeal presence for her in the White House. If Ford could save lives by mobilizing women to examine their breasts and get mammograms, other obstacles could be tackled.

In order to provide a historically accurate framework, it is important to examine the larger picture of mainstream representations of breast cancer that resulted from her revelation. To accompany the *New York Times* articles on Ford, science writer Jane Brody produced a series laying out in nonscientific English a Cancer 101 course for readers. She wove her medical reporting into the narrative of the first lady's illness. In the first article in this series she teaches readers that prognosis depends on the level of cell advancement into the lymphatic system: "Mrs. Ford's tumor, which her doctors said measured two centimeters (less than one inch) across, was a small, early cancer. It was not detected as recently as seven months ago, when Mrs. Ford was last examined" ("Fast" 23). Her writing assumes that her audience—likely a well-educated, middle-class, and international readership—did not read scientific articles. Learning about breast cancer through a story that riveted women—in a soap opera–like saga—became possible because the editors physically laid the two stories—Ford's and Brody's—side by side each day.

If the daily installments of Ford's story and Brody's reporting did not lure female readers, then perhaps Brody's attempt to scare women into examining their breasts would work. The logic seems skewed, but most reporters published statistics on mortality rates for women with breast cancer for that effect (although these statistics did not specify race or socioeconomic status). In 1974 breast cancer was the most common type of cancer in women in the United States (ninety thousand cases in 1974). Breast cancer was the leading killer of women aged forty to forty-four. In 1974, thirty-three thousand women died of breast cancer. Those producing the mass media articles operated from a belief that they could educate women only by alarming them. Ironically, Brody undercut that strategy when she reported that women's fear of breast cancer hindered their self-examination: "A special Gallup poll last year found that women were more worried about breast cancer than any other disease, but fewer than one in five examines her breasts regularly and only half have an annual breast examination done by a physician" ("Fast" 23). It appears counterintuitive for her to try to frighten women into taking control over their bodies given that she reports that it had inhibited women from doing so in the past. Armed with the power of Ford's mastectomy, however, she struck a chord that seemingly altered women's practices.

Women fell victim to their understandable trepidation of the then-standard procedure, which denied women agency with respect to their bodies when it came to removing their breast(s). As practice dictated,

Ford signed a consent form allowing the doctor to perform a Halsted radical mastectomy (just as Carson had done before her) if pathologists found, during biopsy, that the lump was malignant. The first lady, like other women, did not have an opportunity to choose how her body would be treated. On September 29, 1974, the *New York Times* made this topic a front-page story, complete with a photograph of a beleaguered President Ford above the headline "Ford's Wife Undergoes Breast Cancer Surgery." The story describes Ford's Halsted in ways that camouflaged the radicality of the procedure and the process. The article flatly states the circumstances Ford and all other women endured. The article continues in this vein: "Although she knew that she *might* have to undergo a breast removal, Mrs. Ford was described by aides as in 'really good spirits' when she awoke at 6 A.M. today" (Hunter 22; emphasis added). The report accurately implies that Ford did not know whether she would still have her right breast when she woke up. It did not, however, convey the emotional difficulties women suffered as a result of a barbaric surgery and a lack of agency in their medical procedures.

Tragically, two days after Ford's surgery, the NCI released findings from a nationwide study stating that the Halsted radical mastectomy offered no advantage over a less mutilating procedure ("Breast" 26). The *New York Times* printed this report opposite its story on her recovery. The article appeared without any critique of—or thought given to—the fact that Ford (like millions of other women) never had the opportunity to choose her surgery. Because of the archaic procedure forcing women to sign their rights away at the time of biopsy, alternatives based on new scientific developments like this one remained far removed from hospital practices. Through her misfortune Ford became an icon of women's impotence in the medical arena, and this representation of her helped the media to teach women about their surgical options. Reporters took advantage of the first lady's story to publicize why women needed to have a voice in their health care.

One of the most important facets of Brody's investigation was her discovery of discrepancies in surgical research. Because of the cosmetic and emotional scars of mastectomy, she used her column to analyze the data in ways that would assist readers in determining how much surgery a woman actually needed (depending on the particulars of her case) to recover from the disease. Brody also unveiled another, suppressed, alternative to mastectomy known as lumpectomy. Yet she explained that most doctors ignored lumpectomy as a viable option for some patients; the one exception to this rule, Crile, is noticeably absent from the article. The brewing surgical controversy chronicled in the *New York Times* accentuated the care and treatment of cancer patients, although, tellingly, it did not highlight the race- and class-based inequities that were equally problematic. Women's breasts—despite or indeed because of their mass cultural fetishization—were surgically removed without any regard to women's role in making that decision. Primarily white, male medical practitioners decided what type of surgery would stop breast cancer from spreading. Women did not have an opportunity to examine other surgical possibilities, nor were they informed that a biopsy and a mastectomy could be separate procedures. Brody's writing worked in tandem with representations of Ford's experience to teach women how to exercise some control. But the limitations of journalism prevented her from overtly trying to persuade surgeons to change their practices.

Brody's lack of personal experience, in addition to her position as an objective reporter, restricted her from launching a full-scale attack on the medical establishment. Judy Klemesrud took a different approach, concentrating on the emotional scars of less prominent women. Deviating from her peers, she credited Shirley Temple Black's and Marvella Bayh's public announcements almost two years earlier with introducing breast cancer into public discourse ("After" 46).[16] Klemesrud's article appeared in the "Family, Food, Fashion, Furnishings" section of the paper—a site undoubtedly chosen for its targeted female audience. In this specifically feminized section of the newspaper the article invites private female citizens to share their breast cancer experiences too. Felski argues that feminist confession depends on an encoded female audience "marked by . . . a focus upon subjectivity and a construction of identity which is communal rather than individualistic" (115). Clearly this analysis aptly applies to Klemesrud's decision to write about ordinary women with breast cancer. The impetus to feature private citizens demonstrates how Ford's story motivated some people to join forces by acknowledging their membership in a burgeoning and vocal group of women with breast cancer. In the pages of the newspaper where one expects to find photographs of women in the latest fashions, a story about breast cancer ostensibly captured female readers.

Klemesrud's article was one of the first to look at breast cancer as it affected women of color and working-class women, an effort on her part to unify their stories and struggles. Some of the less prominent patients she concentrated on—Adrienne Johnson, a twenty-one-year-old black secretary, and Ann Winkler, a thirty-nine-year-old white artist—cited the silence around breast cancer and the dreaded loss of femininity as the most devastating issues. In the article these women appear healthy in their close-up head shots. Klemesrud also alleviated worries of readers by presenting the women's accounts of their husbands and boyfriends, who did not make them feel any less feminine or desirable without their breasts. The article closes with Bayh's promise of being able to wear low-cut evening gowns despite radical mastectomies—just in case the reader forgot she was reading a story in the fashion pages.

Although Klemesrud's article featured a diverse perspective on breast cancer in terms of race and class, it did not perform the same cultural work in terms of sexuality. As was common for the time, she fixed a heterosexual model of femininity and sexuality to the subject of breast cancer. For example, she highlighted the work of Terese Lasser, whose diagnosis of breast cancer in 1951 led her to found the Reach to Recovery program of the ACS in 1953.[17] Lasser's program deals with the sexual and emotional issues accompanying women's fears about breast cancer. Elucidating the commonplace heterosexist consciousness in the dominant public discourse about breast cancer, Lasser revealed: "'The first thing you think about is whether or not you're going to live. . . . And then the second thing you think about is how the man in your life is going to react'" (Klemesrud, "After," 46). This sentiment plagued novelist Jacqueline Susann, who never confessed to having the disease, nor did she survive it. Klemesrud quoted Susann's husband, Irving Mansfield, who stated that his wife feared her mastectomy because she thought he would leave her.[18] Unlike Ford, many women rooted their feelings about breast cancer in their desirability—sexually and maternally. Lasser's comments focused on life, lived out in the body as well as with the body of the man she lay next to each night.

Obviously breast cancer cannot erase differences with respect to race, class, or sexuality. However, nearly all the reporting, as was standard for the time, focused on an unnamed, middle-class, white audience. Klemesrud's article was one of the first to address, name, or depict these differences at all in the mainstream media. Although black periodicals like *Ebony* also used Ford's announcement as a way to teach its female readers about breast cancer, the mainstream press refrained from widely covering African American singer Minnie Ripperton's breast cancer story two years later.[19] In many of these articles, writers used an approach similar to Brody's, attempting to lessen fear by featuring it prominently as a common emotion all women face. Klemesrud's article begins, "It's been called 'the operation that women fear most' and last Saturday, it was performed on the wife of the President of the United States, Betty Ford" (Klemesrud, "After," 46).

READING THE FIRST LADY'S BODY

Ford's particular style of candor shaped public debates about breast cancer in general and about women's bodies in particular. Sidonie Smith provides a particularly useful way to analyze the subject of female embodiment as it figures into women's autobiography. She argues that embodiment "mark[s] woman with congeries of meaning. If the topography of the universal subject locates man's selfhood somewhere between the ears, it locates woman's selfhood between her thighs. The material and symbolic boundary of the female body becomes the hymen—that physical screen whose presence signals so much" (12). Although Smith's comparison seems somewhat embellished, the anxiety Ford obfuscates within her postmastectomy body reveals the tension between the invisible and the hypervisible parts of women's bodies, which tend to define them. If women's bodies can derive so much meaning from a transparent physical body part, then by extension breasts as a visible gender and sex marker carry with them an equally fraught subjectivity.[20] The first lady's initial disclosure placed the focus on her as wounded in a way that resulted in a hyperembodiment of her disease—that is, it often reduced her to her body. Because she lived in the public eye, she most certainly found herself reduced to her body while processing the emotional response to losing her breast. I would argue that such a representation of her is not empowering; yet, the fact that she went public licensed other women to relinquish the stigma attached to mastectomy. She enabled women to openly discuss breast cancer in public, which mediated the dominant cultural anxiety about women's breasts.

Ford altered the way the public viewed women with breast cancer by telling a story with her voice and with her body. In visibly significant ways, the image of her body coupled with her careful rhetoric had a dramatic effect. Arthur Frank provides a meaningful paradigm for this phenomenon. He establishes an imperative for ill people to tell their stories. Moreover, he elucidates the possibility of bodily empowerment by demonstrating the relationship between the body and the text narrating its story: "The story [is] told *through* a wounded body. The stories that ill people tell come out of their bodies. The body sets in motion the need for new stories when its disease disrupts the old stories. The body, whether still diseased or recovered, is simultaneously cause, topic, and instrument of whatever new stories are told. These embodied stories have two sides, one personal and the other social" (2). Put another way, Frank's theory pinpoints the necessity for ill people to create new narratives about themselves and in effect to alter their realities through their use of language. In this respect Ford gave voice to her postmastectomy body and, as Frank suggests, spoke through her body.

Frank posits the two sides of embodied stories; however, the personal and the social are most usefully thought of with respect to Ford by shifting the words to the confessional and the public. Acknowledging Ford's confessional rhetoric as originating in her body is crucial to examining the social and personal as well as the political and public responses to her illness. In the process of refining his argument about bearing witness to embodied stories, Frank applies his analysis to a critique of the commonly used term *survivor* as it typically describes women who live without metastasis for five years. He renames these survivors *witnesses*: "Becoming a witness assumes a responsibility for telling what happened. The witness offers testimony to a truth that is generally unrecognized or suppressed" (2). Frank's passage demonstrates that breast cancer survivors, or witnesses, testify to their experiences both through their bodies and through their narratives. Discussing breast cancer by fusing a confessional model and a model that relies on bearing witness unpacks the rhetorical complexities about audience, writing or speaking style, and the reverberation of public debates. Ford represented herself as a witness through white-glove rhetoric. Although women before, like Black, went public with their breast cancer, their stories did not have the testimonial power of the White House behind them.

The first lady bore witness to her breast cancer by inviting the press to display her recovery in words and pictures. This effort publicized the

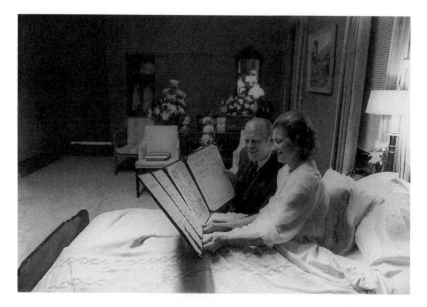

2. Betty and Gerald Ford reading get-well greetings in hospital bed. Courtesy, Gerald R. Ford Library.

disease and offered a daily representation of a public woman with breast cancer on the front page of national newspapers like the *New York Times* and the *Washington Post*. Visually demonstrating the contrast between public and private women, newspapers updated the public on Ford's progress for one week alongside photographs of her in the hospital. These visual representations of her recuperation contributed to the creation of a traditional representation of a middle-class, white wife by showing a woman standing by her man (even though readers might expect the reverse to be true). This portrait took the focus off her postmastectomy body and relieved national anxiety about the president and the first family. One such example shows Ford reading a message, with her husband by her side, from all one hundred senators—the ultimate bourgeois, white, male public (Figure 2). Another photograph depicts Ford playing the ultimate men's sport: throwing a football to her husband with her right arm (a feat nearly impossible for a woman who has just had a Halsted radical mastectomy) (Figure 3). These documents counteracted the anxiety about the debilitating process of healing from a Halsted and the possibility of a husband's being dedicated to his wife's recovery.

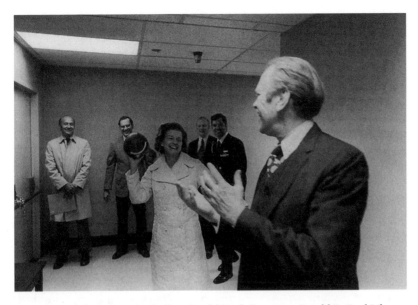

3. Betty Ford throwing a football to Gerald Ford. Courtesy, Gerald R. Ford Library.

But the first lady throwing the football, in a larger context, actually indicated a reinforced traditional femininity. It demonstrated merely that she continued to be a good wife who stood by her husband. Journalist Rose Kushner worried that this front-page, newsworthy gesture worked against Ford as "a well-publicized advertisement for her Halsted radical mastectomy" (*Alternatives* 209). The Halsted drastically disables and reduces the use of a woman's arm for the rest of her life—let alone one week later. Women with mastectomies who saw that image knew how excruciatingly it was for Ford to even lift her arm. Unaware at the time of the political-medical implications of her toss, she characterized it as a simple act demonstrating how diligently she exercised and retrained the remaining strands of her pectoral and arm muscles. Amazingly the Fords described the toss as spontaneous. The president had attended a Washington Redskins football game, and all the players on the team had signed the football for his wife. The story is that when she surprised the president by greeting him at the elevator, he simply threw her gift as a pass, which she caught and threw back to him as public evidence of her healing process.

Ford explains this pivotal moment in her autobiography by framing it in the context of her marriage: "I never felt a psychic wound, I never felt hopelessly mutilated. After all, Jerry and I had been married a good many years, and our love had proved itself. I had no reason to doubt my husband" (205–206). This example of Ford's carefully groomed rhetoric may strike readers as bizarre or out of context in that it seems unconnected to her illness and her recovery—let alone to her football toss—but her logic seems quite common for heterosexual women who face mastectomy. Because many women locate their desirability in their breasts, the loss of a breast anticipates the loss of love. Much like the women in Klemesrud's piece, Ford understood that her feeling about her body depended on her husband's reaction to it. She comforted other women by verifying for them that the loss of a breast did not mean the loss of a marriage. Throwing the football, then, enabled her to visually bear witness to the fact that her body was recovering and that her husband was dealing with her scarred body. Despite the power behind her message it held the potential to convey the sense that her husband was a caring man. On one level Ford encouraged women to face breast cancer in spite of fears about losing a breast or a spouse. On another level she did not challenge the notion that a wounded body could potentially handicap a woman's desirability. However, the visual representations of the first lady proved to be problematic in that they reiterated on a national scale the dangerous myth that breast cancer remained a middle-class, white woman's disease.

The woman who benefited most obviously from Ford's candid, visual, and verbal testimony was Vice President Nelson Rockefeller's wife, Happy. Nineteen days after Ford's surgery, Happy Rockefeller performed a breast self-exam (BSE) and detected a lump "just as countless other women did—after Mrs. Ford's illness received wide publicity" ("Confirmation" 18). Ford remembers watching Nelson Rockefeller speak of his wife on television: "He said . . . that my having told the world I had cancer had helped save Happy's life because it had caused her to go—in time—for a checkup" (211). The reporting of Rockefeller's uncanny coincidence can best be contextualized as being aimed at the dominant public of women who performed BSE and discovered lumps in their breasts. Rockefeller's story unfolded as a result of Ford's: "Like millions of other worried women, Happy Rockefeller reacted to the news of Betty

Ford's breast cancer by giving herself a manual breast examination—even though she had undergone a complete checkup only four months ago. To her dismay she found a lump the size of her finger tip in her left breast" ("Happy's" 29).

One of the stories that began circulating in the media the day immediately following Ford's surgery was that the results of one of Bernard Fisher's early clinical trials, which was begun in 1971, supported Crile's earlier theories that there was no significant difference in outcomes between simple and radical mastectomies ("Breast Cancer Study" 26). The press conference at the NCI had been scheduled prior to Ford's surgery, and her surgeon was aware of these findings, as Barron Lerner illustrates: "[Captain William] Fouty, who performed Ford's surgery and obtained consent from her, knew of this impending announcement. Yet like most surgeons of the era, he continued to believe that a Halsted radical mastectomy was the least risky procedure because the axillary lymph nodes potentially contained cancer. Fouty recommended this operation to Betty and Gerald Ford, although he did mention that some physicians had begun to advocate the use of less extensive surgery" (*Breast Cancer* 172–173). Lerner explains that Ford engaged in a dialogue with her medical team and asked questions that enabled her to participate in the process. It is difficult to know how much the reigning philosophy about the one-step biopsy-mastectomy played into her decision to follow her surgeon's advice. Although Ford may have chosen this standard course of treatment, she might have made a different choice if she, like Rockefeller, had entered the hospital one week after Fisher made his preliminary findings public.

Certainly Rockefeller benefited from the medical questioning in the three weeks between Ford's surgery and her own, as she was able to have a modified radical mastectomy, which saved her chest wall and pectoral muscles.[21] The media opportunity of Ford's and Rockefeller's testimonies and highly publicized surgeries (especially the impact of one on the other) was even greater than when the publicity centered on Ford alone. "With their admirable courage and frankness, Happy Rockefeller and Betty Ford have effected a profound change in the general attitude toward a dread disease. Women are showing a new willingness to discuss breast cancer openly, to face it directly" ("Breast," *Time*, 107).

Ford's and Rockefeller's witnessing to their breast cancer affected women by contributing to public debate and by encouraging women to examine their own bodies through BSE. Reporters described the waiting lists at clinics across the country, clinics that previously received thirty to forty calls became flooded with over four hundred calls daily ("Hectic"; Baker; "Mammography 1982"; Turnbull). Obviously, neither woman could control all of the public response to—or the representations of—her body in the media. Ford gave birth to the public debates about breast cancer, but her story took on a life of its own. Perhaps the most crucial legacy of Ford's limited agency in the rhetorical and visual representations of her body was the forum she provided for complicating the mediated entanglement of her breast-cancered body in a private, personal struggle. To recover in a public setting meant that Ford had to negotiate how she would present her one-breasted body. Because Ford helped to publicize her illness, the media assumed her private body was up for public discussion, scrutiny, and debate. But Ford used her bodily experience as a way to own—and to mediate to some extent—the representations of her body and her illness.

Despite the heightened awareness of feminism and the women's health movement in the 1970s, euphemisms about women's bodies remained firmly entrenched in polite rhetoric. The words *breast cancer* and *mastectomy,* despite their clinical connotations, were as vivid as a photograph of Ford's scarred chest would have been. Her uneasiness about being a public figure related to her middle-class discomfort about presenting herself in public. Specifically, throughout her husband's career Ford constantly struggled with her precarious position as a lady in white gloves. Breast cancer plagued her because it rendered her body hypervisible. It forced her to become overly aware of her body and people's responses to it. On the one hand her visibility promoted the importance of early detection. On the other hand breast cancer became her identity in much the same way her alcoholism later would.

Sharing their private experiences may not have been personally empowering for Ford and Rockefeller, but it ignited other women who read their stories. The combined effect of these narratives proved, as Elspeth Probyn argues, that bodies "negotiat[e] the dominant discourses of their times" (113). As in Ford's case, women's bodies become sites of power when women control the representations of their bodies and their stories. Yet, as Probyn demonstrates, constructing a status grounded in—but not reduced to—the body remains a difficult, if not impossible, prospect. Elizabeth Grosz argues that because bodies are "coded with and as signs" they become "narrativized." She asserts, "If bodies are traversed and infiltrated by knowledges, meanings, and power, they can also, under certain circumstances, become sites of struggle and resistance, actively in-scribing themselves on social practices" (35–36). In other words, for women the body always represents struggle and contradiction, but it holds the potential to disrupt social practices and ways of thinking.

It may be more difficult to find ways to dislodge the way we imagine and portray the subjectivity of women in the spotlight. Ironically, *Time's* cover story for the week of Ford's surgery focused on the public burden political wives bear. The article, which ran with a sidebar story on breast cancer and Ford's recovery, claimed that the ordeal of political wives de-rives from their role as "public property, an extension of the public man, subject to unending scrutiny, judgments, accolades and criticism" (Angelo 15). The rhetoric recalls nineteenth-century separate spheres, when hus-bands and fathers quite literally owned women as property. As Ford blurred the boundaries between public and private, this rhetoric served as a reminder that the public maintained control over representations of women. The photographs of Ford throwing the football to the president and of her reading letters from members of Congress could be thought of in this respect. Not only were those opportunities for her to say "I'm okay" to the public, but President Ford could also make it clear that he was okay as well. In other words, images of public women continued to be contingent on men's public representations.

Ford's illness dominated *Newsweek's* content as well; the magazine ran a close-up photograph of Ford's face on its cover with a two-word caption: "The Operation." By the time the magazine hit newsstands, her predicament was so well known that the words *breast cancer* did not even need to be used. The mastectomy—the operation women fear most—re-mained absent on the cover, although not in the pages, of the magazine. Here, too, the writers emphasized and acknowledged the distinction be-tween private and public and then collapsed it: "Inevitably, the Ford fam-ily's private anguish became a public event" ("Betty" 30). In this article, their personal crisis overshadows the president's political and national problems, such as the economy, the energy crisis, his unpopular pardon of President Nixon, and his offer of amnesty to conscientious objectors of the Vietnam War. In the arena of domestic politics, the first lady's candor about her illness fit into the framework of national political issues, as did also her frank support of the Equal Rights Amendment (ERA), abortion, liberalized marijuana laws, trial marriages, and civil rights.[22] Finally, this article offered hope, as in earlier reporting, with its medical perspectives on the treatable nature of breast cancer and its citing of other famous women who had breast cancer, most notably Alice Roosevelt Longworth, who referred to herself as "'Washington's topless octogenarian'" ("Betty" 30).

Instituting celebrity bodies as tools to convey social practices and new knowledge seemed so extensive that it led *Newsweek* columnist Shana Alexander to mount a backlash: "The tone and volume of reportage on Mrs. Nelson Rockefeller's . . . operation for breast cancer compel one to shout: enough! Enough medical detailing of private matters for public scrutiny" ("Breast" 122).[23] Ironically, Alexander dissects this subject as one that falls into neatly demarcated, dichotomized public and private spheres. Her anxiety about private subjects becoming public debates illustrates, perhaps, a more widespread panic about the embodiment of women and, specifically, about breast cancer. Apparently Ford's white-glove rhetoric does not deceive this reporter. She attempts to regulate the proliferation of the bodily discourse in the media by summoning her peers to return to traditional, ladylike decorum. Ironically, the cultural norms she perpetuates would exclude her from participating in the media. She longs for traditional news stories that obstruct the body from public view. But, historically, sanitized language depended on a white, male author with an abstract body. Decorum may occlude discussion of the body; however, it also excludes any subject whose body figures prominently.

Alarmingly, Alexander leans toward allowing male codes of female public presence to prevail. Her column pleads with public officials to revert to the privacy of their doctor's office when discussing personal matters. In particular she objects to the use of Ford's and Rockefeller's breast cancer to highlight medical research: "This is *news*? What is going on in there, a mastectomy or a hijacking?" Although she knows they willingly chose to use their experiences to educate the public, and she believes their act saved lives, Alexander takes issue with "a certain harshness of language and obsession with clinical detail." Words like "removing a cancerous left breast" coming from the mouths of anchors on the nightly news or from reporters in the pages of the magazine she works for strike her as "unnecessarily specific and unpleasant" ("Breast" 122). She remains trapped in a dominant—indeed misogynist—logic. And yet she positions herself in her editorial as a citizen, a woman, and a prospective patient given the then-current statistics pointing to breast cancer as the leading killer of women in the United States. All her annoyed ranting leads me to wonder whether her desire to repress breast cancer came from the same fear the first and second ladies' testimonies unraveled. Alexander's response was in some respects classic repression: she clearly wanted to silence these images and issues yet at the same time she could not stop talking about them, a contradiction that ultimately revealed her own anxiety and ambivalence.

Alexander complains of news overkill, especially with respect to medical information, but her column contributes to it. Moreover, she contradicts herself when she criticizes confessions about women's bodies and women's health—tales that clearly fascinated her: "Everyone is confessing everything—medical records, bank accounts, psychiatric despairs, sexual kinks, all manner of bleeding wounds and running sores of the spirit are on show or on sale. Some mass urge to confess, to display, to fling off aprons seems to be epidemic. Decorum, seemliness, all respect for privacy of person appear to have been tossed aside in the mania to take it *all* off, to tell it like it is, to—most hideous usage!—let it all hang out" ("Breast" 122).[24] Her trepidation prompted her to reach back to a 1950s mentality, in which the distinction between public and private remained rigid and codes of decorum magically made middle-class white ladies stand silently by their men. Perhaps some of her angst accumulated over time. Confessions of public officials during Watergate characterized the political and discursive climate of the early 1970s. The impulse to neatly cover up what Alexander deemed intrinsically private eventually led Ford, Rockefeller, and countless other women who followed suit to confess in public. But Alexander maintained that baring all is inappropriate behavior for ladies who wear white gloves.

LIMITATIONS AND MANIPULATIONS OF FORD'S CONFESSION

A white postmastectomy woman's body in the mass media presented a conundrum. Ford's body perpetuated a dangerous myth that breast cancer primarily afflicts white, middle-class, heterosexual women. The statistical truth hidden beneath this perception was that although fewer black women were diagnosed with breast cancer, mortality rates for African American women were—and remain—significantly higher than those for white women (Bassett and Krieger 1401). Mary Bassett and Nancy Krieger's study reveals that in the time just prior to Ford's disclosure, and for the next decade, "at the time of diagnosis, Black and White breast cancer patients differed in three respects: Blacks were younger than Whites, had more advanced disease, and were of poorer social class standing" (1401). Moreover, NCI data suggest that between 1974 and 1976 white women had a 75 percent relative survival rate while black women had a 62 percent relative survival rate. One of the reasons for the disparities contained in these numbers could be William McWhorter and William Mayer's finding that "Black patients were more likely than Whites to be untreated . . . and to be treated by non-surgical methods" (1516). One plan that purported to change these statistics was the BCDDP, which screened women for breast cancer through mammography, a system for detecting tumors before they became malignant.[25] The program was designed to screen all women—especially those with limited economic means—in clinics set up across the country. Although the NCI and ACS detection program attempted to extinguish the disparity between black and white women's mortality rates from breast cancer, if African American women did not receive the same treatment postdiagnosis—especially if their diagnosis came at a late stage of the disease—the screening program would have only a slight effect.

Representations of Ford's illness in the mass media encouraged thousands of women to go to the BCDDP clinics. Seemingly overnight she became the spokeswoman for the NCI and ACS effort to teach BSE and to screen women regularly through mammography at its clinics. Ford's support inadvertently assisted the NCI and the ACS with the BCDDP, a program waiting for a publicity angle to attract the mass media and a mass public. She epitomized a presentable (read: white lady) celebrity, and this representation enabled her to convince the public that mammography could detect lumps early. Although she struggled with confronting the contested meanings surrounding her hypervisible body, she recognized her enormous potential to educate women about breast cancer. But like the many paradoxes that followed, this pedagogical project became more complicated than simply claiming control of her own representation. With or without her support the NCI and the ACS appropriated her image and her story to publicize its program and its clinics.

The NCI officials running the BCDDP were not nearly as candid or as public about the relative risks of radiation from mammography as Ford had been about her operation. The risks were especially great for young women, whose breasts were more susceptible to the rays. The BCDDP annual reports do not mention any such risks and are equally evasive about the reason (i.e., Betty Ford's breast cancer) their program turned out to be successful (i.e., they had many women screened). Ostensibly today mammograms can be a useful way to screen postmenopausal women because the level of radiation is regulated; in the 1970s they were hazardous and arguably carcinogenic.[26] Appallingly, the NCI, the ACS, and the ACR knew during the time of the BCDDP operation that for some women mammography led to a high risk of obtaining cancer. Samuel Epstein chronicles the "large-scale routine screening of premenopausal women in the 1970s" in which the NCI, the ACS, and the ACR admitted knowing these alarming facts (351). Furthermore, Epstein explains that although "mammography in women over the age of 50 could lead to a reduction in mortality of breast cancer by 30 to 50 percent . . . mammography in younger women . . . is associated with increased risks of breast cancer, which may balance possible diagnostic advantages" (313).

Placing the decision to get a mammogram in women's hands ultimately proved to be counterproductive. It entrenched a blame-the-victim approach, making women responsible for detecting cancer in their bodies. Moreover, in a study evaluating the BCDDP program, researchers conceded that the women who volunteered to be screened tended to be "more highly educated, above average socioeconomically, and both healthy and health conscious; in addition, they were concerned about breast cancer, symptomatic, or at higher risk" (Smart et al. 144). Thus, when the BCDDP redirected Ford's media attention to promote its clinics, it did not necessarily attract working-class women or women of color; this result illustrates the limits of the first lady's agency, and it also suggests the limits of such programs in trying to attract a wide variety of women who may or may not take advantage of the affordable and promising technology in free clinics. In fact, retrospective studies demonstrate that, between 1950 and 1992, "breast cancer mortality rates for white women were relatively stable" and "breast cancer mortality rates for black women increased over time" (Flaws, Newschaffer, and Bush 1008).

Moreover, as Patricia Kaufert illustrates, "while many U.S. physicians were taught during the 1980s that lives were to be saved by screening, some also learned that money was to be made" (175).[27] Hence, just as past surgical practices were institutionalized based on the profits to be made by cutting away large portions of the breast, the screening and detection program was never only about saving lives. This subversion of the intentions of the screening program again illustrates the limits of the first lady's agency: this complicated and subtle understanding of the screening process did not get communicated to the public.

At the time, the NCI and the ACS used BSE as a strategy for "preventing" breast cancer, and they promoted mammography technology in the same way. But neither was "preventative." They gave women an important sense of control over their bodies but also a false sense of security (or alarm) as the case may be. One example is the pointed narrative Rockefeller published in *Reader's Digest*, where she pleaded with readers to see their doctors if they suspected a lump: "Don't waste time on disbelief. Find out. *And don't be afraid!* If you must have surgery, remember: it is not as horrible as you think it's going to be; the anticipation is the hardest part" (134). Rockefeller opened the narrative by insisting she wanted to retell her story—to bear witness to her body's experience—because "my story can help alert—and encourage—others" to practice BSE as she had (131). To know one's body, and one's breasts, enables women to ascertain the difference between abnormal and normal lumps. But to rely entirely on BSE to the exclusion of clinical breast exams and mammograms can be detrimental. Moreover, none of these practices—even when combined—prevents breast cancer. Herein lies another limitation of Ford's and Rockefeller's agency: this complicated and crucial understanding of the screening process did not get communicated to the public. An article by Brody in the *New York Times* ("Inquiries" 21), for example, mistakenly equated detection with prevention, perhaps leading many women to believe mammography could "prevent" breast cancer when the technology more likely caused it.

As this chapter illustrates, intense interest in Ford's body—which culminated in more women engaging with their bodies—correlated with the way her body and voice figured prominently in the media. Although Ford's confession about her breast cancer diagnosis effectively empowered other women with breast cancer, it is not so clear that Ford experienced similar gains for herself. Nancy Fraser warns that "it is not correct to view publicity as always and unambiguously an instrument of empowerment and emancipation. For members of subordinate groups, it will always be a matter of balancing potential political uses of publicity against the dangers of loss of privacy" ("Sex" 332). The first lady took conventional codes of self-representation and reworked them for less conventional ends, while the media, the ACS, and the NCI manipulated her public image for their own purposes. Ford's and Rockefeller's candid confessions produced a forum for public debate about women's agency over their bodies in the medical arena—a debate that ultimately facilitated Rose Kushner's abolition of the one-step biopsy–radical mastectomy. Ford helped to increase awareness about breast cancer in the mass media, even as the NCI and the ACS capitalized on her publicity for its promotion of its dangerous mammography campaign. Nonetheless, as the first public spokeswoman and icon for breast cancer survival in the United States, Ford reached a wide audience with her white-glove confessional rhetoric and encouraged women to take control of their lives and their bodies.

CHAPTER 3

Rose Kushner versus the
Medical Establishment

DEFENDING A WOMAN'S
RIGHT TO CHOOSE

IN THE FALL of 1974 Betty Ford's and Happy Rocke-
feller's public disclosures about their breast cancer ended a silence that
forced women before them to suffer in private. From their stories and the
mass media's representations of their stories, the public learned a great
deal about cancer and scientific advances in oncology treatment and
screening practices.[1] Although the overwhelming body of material circulated through the print and visual media appeared to release breast cancer
from the silence that had surrounded it, a reticence to tackle the issues
that the first and second ladies' illnesses illuminated remained. One of the
primary aspects the media illuminated was that Ford had not participated
in deciding what type of treatment she would have. On hearing of Ford's
plans for a one-step Halsted radical mastectomy, Rose Kushner, the first
breast cancer activist in the United States, attempted to intervene in
Ford's biopsy and surgery. She tried to deliver a message to President Ford
through one of his speechwriters, Milton Friedman. Kushner wanted the
first lady to know she could wait to have her operation and choose a less
mutilating surgery. The speech writer responded to Kushner by saying,
" 'I am sorry. The President has made *his* decision.' "[2] Angered by this response, Kushner used this anecdote when she tried to place in *Ms.* magazine a breast cancer article detailing the "male-chauvinist-piggery"
inherent in the lack of agency available to women with breast cancer.

Kushner may not have been able to reach Ford, but countless other
women, including Rockefeller, heard her voice when she published an
article in the *Washington Post* about choices available to women confronted with breast cancer. In fact, it appears that Rockefeller benefited

directly. After hearing a rumor that Rockefeller chose a modified surgery based on that article, Kushner wrote a letter to the second lady. In it she alluded to this connection: "When I learned that you, like Mrs. Ford, had become a member of Mrs. [Alice] Longworth's mastectomy club, I immediately wondered if you had been helped by reading this story. Your decision to have a modified-radical instead of a Halsted-radical . . . coming so soon after publication seemed to be more than a coincidence."[3] Arguably, Rockefeller's decision came out of a variety of news reports released beginning the day after Ford's surgery. A distinct cause-and-effect line cannot be traced between Kushner's article and Rockefeller's choice. However, the media fervor surrounding these political wives provided Kushner with an audience of women whom she empowered to make decisions about their bodies.

On some level the publicity in the mass media raised Kushner's awareness of the pedagogical potential of the press. She indicated that such authority seemed reserved for political celebrities, and yet she also participated in public debates about breast cancer. This realization helped her to envision writing a book about breast cancer as a consciousness-raising vehicle for women. In the book she explained the situation before Ford's and Rockefeller's disclosures when she was diagnosed with breast cancer:

> Of course, everyone in Washington knew about Alice Longworth, Theodore Roosevelt's astonishing daughter. She had had both her breasts removed for cancer almost a half century ago and billed herself as "the flattest-chested woman in the capital." Sometimes she joked that she was the only really topless woman in town. But former presidents' daughters are legends; that's why she survived. Mere mortal women died from breast cancer. Betty Ford and Happy Rockefeller had not yet discovered their tumors. The flood of information and optimistic facts that filled newspapers and magazines after their operations had not yet appeared. There was nothing I had ever come across to show me anything but the shadow of imminent death. (*Alternatives* 1–2)

This description of the climate in which she found out about her illness reminds us of a universe more akin to the one in which Rachel Carson discovered that she had breast cancer. Although Carson was a celebrity in Washington circles in the early 1960s, she also was a mere mortal woman who did not survive the disease. Silence about breast cancer did not just mean keeping it hidden from the public as Ford's example illustrates. Silence about breast cancer also can be gleaned from the lack of reporting on the subject in the dominant public sphere.

When the intense spotlight surrounding the first and second ladies dimmed, attention turned to some not-so-famous women, like Rose Kushner, who found their voices by publishing memoirs or self-help manuals about breast cancer. These texts extended public discourse about breast cancer by mediating the larger consciousness-raising project initiated by Ford. In this chapter I examine one such book, *Breast Cancer: A Personal History and an Investigative Report,* written by Kushner.[4] This self-help book was the first breast cancer book written by someone who bore witness to the illness with the intention of educating women about their bodies and the medical system. Capitalizing on what she saw as the first lady's impotence when it came to making decisions about how her body would be treated, Kushner taught women how to access the necessary information to facilitate having a voice in their healthcare.

It is often difficult to confirm a definitive relationship between a text and the effect it has on public culture. But the historical time in which Kushner wrote lends itself to this type of reading. Building on the momentum of a public craving accessible information about breast cancer, she altered perceptions and shifted debates about mastectomy in multiple and at times competing public spheres; she did so not only in print but also, eventually, before Congress. One of the things that paved the way for her political endeavors was 1970s feminist discourse, which provided a model for politically charged writing and which encouraged women to make the private public and the personal political. In her writing and public witnessing Kushner intervened discursively in public debates regarding breast cancer in two groundbreaking ways: first, she created a space for women's agency by struggling to allow women the right to a two-step biopsy and surgery; and, second, she pressured the medical establishment to offer women surgical choices and to outlaw the Halsted radical mastectomy. By using Kushner as an example, this chapter describes the specific movement from breast cancer as a silenced subject to one that gets debated in a public legal sphere and, in so doing, demonstrates how aspects of the consciousness-raising narrative provided the mechanism for this advancement.

BECOMING AN EXPERT WITNESS

Rose Kushner aspired to be a creative writer, but a lack of talent prevented her from finding a publisher for anything beyond a few, nominal journalistic feature stories. She worked as a freelance medical writer, contributing stories on topics such as Tay-Sachs disease, and as a journalist covering the Arab/Israeli War of 1973 and the Vietnam War.[5] Initially her articles appeared primarily in U.S. Jewish newspapers. When she first discovered her name in the *Washington Post,* she was the subject and not the author of articles with headlines like "A Housewife Goes to War." When she was recovering in the hospital from her mastectomy, she seized the opportunity to write the most candid exposé of women's lack of agency in the mastectomy process and their lack of knowledge about surgical options. In a letter to a friend, Kushner reported that it took the *Washington Post* from August 23rd until October 6th to publish her first article: "The tug of war went on until I finally said they should send it back so I could try elsewhere. It took the First Lady to win my battle for me."[6]

Because of her attempt to have agency in her own treatment Kushner had already done all the work that the mass media later did for the public. She researched the disease, its treatments—standard and alternative—and she shared her findings with other patients, doctors, and lawmakers. She published her conclusions in newspapers, women's magazines, feminist health books, an American Cancer Society (ACS) brochure, and three different editions of her book published between 1975 and 1984.[7] In the *Washington Post* article Kushner clearly spelled out for readers that "in most instances a woman going to sleep for a simple biopsy does not know whether she will wake up with one breast or two." Moreover, she questioned this process by pointedly asking: "Why do surgeons feel they have the right to make the decision for their unconscious patients? Why not allow them to wake up, be told the diagnosis and the alternatives and options available?" Her words—which appeared in a section far removed from the editorial pages—represented the lone voice in the mass media advocating for women's agency in their medical care.

Unlike other reporters at the time, Kushner delineated the pressing concerns for women facing a breast cancer diagnosis, and she supported her claims with the latest scientific data. By explaining the biopsy and pathology procedures she alerted her audience to the outdated one-step biopsy and mandatory Halsted. She broke journalistic boundaries by advising women to choose their own operation. In her most feminist voice she asked in her *Washington Post* article, "Why should the doctor, husband, father, brother or whoever make the choice? It is, after all, the woman's life—not theirs." For one of the first times in such a widely circulated periodical, with painstaking detail and in lay language, Kushner carefully listed and explained each of the five medically viable breast surgeries: partial (when the lump and surrounding tissue are removed); simple or total (when the breast is removed but the axillary nodes and chest wall and muscles remain); subcutaneous (when the breast tissue is removed and a silicone implant replaces it); modified-radical (when the breast and axillary nodes are removed with a smaller incision but the muscles and chest wall remain intact); and the Halsted-radical (when the breast, chest wall, axillary nodes, and pectoral muscles are removed). She warned readers about the struggles she confronted. But for women with the time, financial means, and determination she outlines a legible map for taking charge of their medical treatment. In this respect, Kushner's writing deviated from Ford's white-glove rhetoric and altered the perception in the dominant public of brave women catching footballs only a few days after a Halsted.

The overwhelming response to Kushner's brief article in the *Washington Post* revealed the need for women with breast cancer to share not only their illness narratives with the public but also their knowledge about the disease and about doctors as well. In this way, Kushner provided a patients' perspective while facilitating public debates about a patient's right to choose her course of treatment. She extended that discussion in her book *Breast Cancer*, this time enticing readers by folding elements of a traditional memoir into a scientifically researched reference book on breast cancer epidemiology, history, surgery, chemotherapy, radiotherapy, and politics. Rather than relying solely on the personal narrative form, she uses a pedagogical framework to teach women that the personal is political. In many respects Kushner's work embodies the sophisticated definition of that dictum, which Zillah Eisenstein updates:

"The personal has political meaning and political meanings are personally lived. . . . Sexual politics breaks open the public/private divide. However, this insight can be too solipsistic. To say that the personal *is* political
reduces each to the other. To say that the political *is* personal oversimpli-
fies the individualism of politics. But neither is it true that the personal is
not political; or the political is not personal" (41). Kushner may not have
written her book with this nuanced understanding of what a certain
strain of feminist politics entails, but her work and life give us evidence
of the ways in which breast cancer affects women in a politically personal way. From the moment she discovered the barriers to selecting her
own course of treatment, she envisioned sharing this process with the
public. She may not have always imagined herself doing inherently feminist work, but her practices certainly can be viewed as modeling the dictum that the personal is political.

Her books, *Breast Cancer, Why Me?*, and *Alternatives,* construct a systemic, politicized critique and analysis of the medical system and, in
turn, shed light on the ways that women experience oppression in that
context. To attract a wide audience to *Breast Cancer,* she moved seamlessly
from a description of her personal experience with breast cancer into an
explanation of the biology of the disease written in succinct lay terms.
The juxtaposition of these aspects of the disease enabled—and indeed
encouraged—readers to experience a shift in perspective. Simply put,
reading Kushner's narrative raised the consciousness of the reader. Early
second-wave feminist texts provide steps politically minded women can
take to proceed in their communities with consciousness-raising and political work. On this list first and foremost is "reading, analyzing, [and]
writing literature" (Koedt, Levine, and Rapone 280). Consciousness-
raising literature suggests, then, that there is a dialogic relationship between the reader and the text. Writers of this subgenre hope—and indeed anticipate—that readers will act after finishing the text. In other
words, according to Lisa Hogeland, the consciousness-raising genre is
"the process by which participants come to see the personal as political"
(ix). Kushner's writing and the reception of her text can be understood
in this context.

In the emerging subgenre of breast cancer literature, as Ellen
Leopold points out, narratives from the 1970s "were memoirs with a
mission, front-line dispatches, [but] the breast cancer literature that has

emerged since the 1970s has been based more on the Betty Ford template than on the Rose Kushner one. It has turned inward, becoming ever more introspective and idiosyncratic" (*A Darker* 251). In other words, although most memoirs narrated stories that needed to be heard, few of them moved women into action in the way that Kushner's text did. In all three editions of *Breast Cancer*, she documented the process of challenging restrictive codes; and, by speaking about verboten subjects in public forums, she lured even conservative ladies to join her in the public sphere.

The progression of Kushner's story from finding her lump to choosing her treatment provides women with a model of how to act, first in a medical setting and second in a political one. She first discovered a lump in her left breast by accident on June 15, 1974, in the privacy of her shower as she shaved her armpit. She was not doing a breast self-exam (BSE). Although mainstream women's magazines at the time periodically included articles about BSE, the practice did not become somewhat normalized until the third edition of Kushner's book *Alternatives*.[8] In the early 1970s, she reminds her readers, women did not think or talk about breast cancer until the first lady's public disclosure. The timing of her discovery was unfortunate: it was only three months before Ford's breast cancer, and yet that gap in time meant Kushner did not have a diverse set of informational resources available to her. This middle-class, Jewish, feminist journalist from a Maryland suburb of Washington, D.C., found the obstacles to learning about her illness immense: "There was nothing in bookstores or the public library, and I had to go to the library of the National Institutes of Health (NIH) for help" (*Alternatives* xii).

Kushner empowered herself as an active participant in her medical journey. She asserted herself by informing her doctor she would allow only a breast specialist or an oncologist to perform her biopsy. Her doctor responded with astonishment—particularly because he did not expect his patients to know what an oncologist was let alone to ask for one. Amazingly, just minutes away from the NCI in Bethesda, Maryland, he told her, "I don't know of any oncologist in this area who specializes in breasts" (quoted in *Alternatives* 4–5). Perhaps her internist was surprised by her request because at that time general surgeons also performed a variety of specialty surgeries. Still, Kushner refused to take no for an answer. She bravely argued with her physicians at each stage of the process.

Her determination was as heroic as it was rare. At that time breast cancer patients had to fight two wars (the war in their bodies and the war with their doctors) if they wanted any agency over their treatment. Eventually her research paid off because she learned enough about breast cancer to discern her own physical situation. After her first NCI visit she told her husband, "Nobody's hacking off my breast while I'm unconscious unless I'm convinced that that's the only thing there is to do" (*Alternatives* 8). Unbeknownst to her at the time, this informal, private assertion to her husband would catapult her into the center of a very public, political arena.

One book in particular facilitated Kushner's excursion into the dominant public—the only book in the library under the subject heading *breast cancer*. The book was George Crile's *What Women Should Know about the Breast Cancer Controversy*.[9] She initially responded to his text by exclaiming: "I hadn't even known, then, that there *was* a breast-cancer controversy!" (*Alternatives* 9). She and her husband reacted to Crile's book in two contradictory ways. At first they appreciated that he offered a standpoint on the opposite end of the spectrum from currently established norms: empower the woman to choose her own surgery and conserve the breast if at all possible. Later, despite the fact that they wanted to hear this unusual perspective, they perceived him as someone who held a grudge, which in their eyes intimated he was biased and could not be trusted. Kushner reports her husband's concern: "'He [Crile] doesn't write like a scientist. He sounds as if he's on some kind of a vendetta because his wife died even though she had her breast taken off.' 'He does sound bitter about that,' I agreed, 'because it was done for nothing. She went through all the pain and mutilation of a mastectomy, and the cancer had already been spreading'" (*Alternatives* 10). Rose Kushner objected to his writing style partially because the medical reporter in her found his strategy entirely too subjective. Ironically, she had scoured the country for a surgeon who would permit her to participate in the decision-making process, yet once she found that viewpoint, she objected to it. Crile's model advocated women's agency, but Kushner found herself unable to trust the model because of Crile's candor. Regardless of the skew she and her husband detected in Crile's work, the Kushners found solace in learning about alternative surgeries and the accompanying survival rates. Their initial reaction to his writing thus did not last, but it speaks more generally to an expectation that physicians should be objective and distanced from their subjects. At that time it was unusual for a doctor to write a book marketed to the general public; but it was unheard of for a doctor to also divulge his private life and admit that it influenced his medical opinions. Kushner's derisive critique seems inconsistent as she too employs the same rhetoric, tone, tactics, and techniques in her text that she finds troubling in his.

In her research, guided largely by Crile's book, Kushner uncovered the one-step biopsy and mastectomy. This practice outraged Kushner the most; she characterizes the lack of time for processing the emotional ramifications of the procedure and women's lack of agency in the treatment as "barbaric!" (*Alternatives* 12). However, she concedes that some circumstances necessitate a simultaneous biopsy and mastectomy. For instance, if the patient poses a surgical risk, it makes sense to perform only one operation. Also, she acknowledges, some women prefer for psychological and emotional reasons to have one operation rather than two. The standard biopsy process in June 1974 was to fast-freeze the lump, slice it open, and look at it under a microscope to diagnose the patient within a matter of minutes. Sometimes, although rarely, this procedure was not as accurate as more sustained, lengthier pathological testing, and as a result some women had their breasts removed unnecessarily because of misdiagnosis.

Learning about the one-step biopsy and surgery motivated Kushner to become an agent of change. While recovering from her modified radical mastectomy, she began to formulate a link between her private experience and changes that would benefit other women with breast cancer. Her writing originated within a counterpublic community of breast cancer patients but later reverberated in the dominant public, thereby raising the consciousness of lay citizens and legislators. Her work exemplifies Nancy Fraser's articulation of the discursive possibilities in a counterpublic sphere: "Insofar as these counterpublics emerge in response to exclusions within the dominant publics, they help expand discursive space" ("Rethinking" 15). Fraser contends that widening political debates in a stratified society is crucial because it can make a marginalized concern a public one. Kushner's writing eventually led to her becoming an expert witness, providing testimony before Congress; it also opened doors such as opportunities to publish in medical journals, and through these various venues she changed medical practices and public perception in precisely the way Fraser lays out.

Kushner employed a variety of war analogies to explain the basic biology of cancer in her book. She introduces this strategy by telling a story about her experience as a reporter in Vietnam. She recalls attending a press conference in 1967 in which Major Vung Tau described his country's war as analogous to cancer. She quotes his extended metaphor: "'To me, an insurgent is like a fragment of cancer in a healthy body—invading, destroying, and drawing its nourishment from the healthy organs around it. The goal of this fragment of cancer is not to live peacefully side by side; its goal is to replace all the healthy organs with the disease. Its aim is the total destruction of the body—in the case of a nation, the government'" (*Alternatives* 36). Ironically, she writes, she never imagined that she would return to the intersection of Vietnam and cancer. At the time she found Tau's link novel and borrowed it to describe the war to her readers in the United States. She revisits this description and inverts it in her book on breast cancer: "A human body invaded by cancer is like a country battling a small guerrilla insurgency. If the government (body) is strong and healthy, if there are no weak spots in its society (possible genetic predisposing factors), if there are no traitors within the government to help the enemy (chemical, viral, or radiation carcinogens), and if the defense machinery (the immunological system) is strong, then the insurgency can be put down with a minimum of over-all damage. A microscopic cancerous rebellion, started in the proper environment and supported and nourished by various contributing factors, can grow and grow, until—like the war in Vietnam—it endangers the very life of the whole body" (*Alternatives* 37). Kushner does not comment on her use of Vietnam to depict a devastating disease. She merely invokes it as an illustrative way to explain cancer in the simplest terms, terms she believed would resonate most profoundly in her readers. Moreover, as a journalist, Kushner wanted to inform her audience without analyzing the data or critiquing her own methodology.

After the one-step biopsy and Halsted radical mastectomy were eradicated, Kushner continued to find ways to improve women's treatment in the healthcare setting. Almost ten years after her diagnosis, she began to draw analogies between overzealous surgery and chemotherapy. Arguing that the excessive use of chemotherapy resembled the overuse of the Halsted radical mastectomy prior to Betty Ford, she writes about the continuing practice of not allowing women to have a choice about how to treat their bodies. In an essay entitled "Is Aggressive Adjuvant Chemotherapy the Halsted Radical of the '80s?" she addressed these concerns to oncologists in the journal *CA: A Cancer Journal for Clinicians*. Although some of her claims are a bit out of date, many of them remain critical. Her primary concern was the continuing lack of attention to the patient's emotional and physical well-being; she argued, "In the United States, baldness, nausea and vomiting, diarrhea, clogged veins, financial problems, broken marriages, disturbed children, loss of libido, loss of self-esteem, and body image are nurse's turf" (345).[10] In other words, because a gendered and hierarchical system of care exists in most hospitals, the work of assisting patients with side effects from chemotherapy typically falls on the shoulders of nurses. Typically doctors do not witness the bulk of the difficulties of coping with chemotherapy. Therefore, chemotherapy's toxic effects remain hidden from or ignored by oncologists; they concern themselves with increasing the woman's quantity of life often to the detriment of her quality of life.

This discrepancy is particularly unsettling because the results of an NCI study, published the same year as Kushner's article, revealed that, of sixty thousand breast cancer patients tracked between 1973 and 1980, "those who were given only a single course of cytotoxic chemotherapy had more than eight times the relative risk of developing acute nonlymphocytotic leukemia within three years after treatment, as did the women who had not received the drugs" ("Is Aggressive" 349).[11] Thus, thirty-one years after these cancer-fighting drugs were discovered, they continued to have a toxic effect that did not necessarily cure cancer nor did they definitively increase the patient's life span. Instead, these drugs, which are increasingly used in an adjuvant (precautionary treatment to reduce the likelihood that the cancer will spread) setting, dramatically interfere with the patient's quality (and possibly quantity) of life.

Leopold maintains that Kushner's significance is unmatched: "Kushner's book was really the first attempt to use a personal narrative of breast cancer as a springboard to a much broader discussion. A memoir, a comprehensive handbook, and a manifesto all rolled into one, it opened up an extraordinarily rich debate" (*A Darker* 234). Kushner's narrative style effectively drew several different audiences at once. Women with breast cancer read and benefited from her candid information about treatment. And if they could afford it, they used her book to help them find doctors who would listen to them. As women began to rely on her book, they brought it to the attention of their doctors. As studies from the medical community increasingly corroborated the claims Kushner made to the lay public, her voice reached wider audiences, including the offices on Capitol Hill.

A HOUSEWIFE GOES TO CONGRESS

Whether she wrote for a clinical or a mainstream public audience, Kushner made clear her concerns about women's lives; this impassioned style of writing gave way to her activism and eventually her activism provided her with different venues for publishing. In some ways, her value lies more in her role as an activist than as a writer, although writing was a vehicle for publicizing her political goals.[12]

Initially, Kushner did not anticipate that her skepticism of surgical practices would lead her to a crusade to abolish the one-step biopsy and mastectomy. And yet her role as an expert witness ultimately led to the mandate that doctors separate the two procedures in order to alleviate psychological repercussions and to allow women to get a second opinion. After reconciling her feelings about Crile, she eventually shared a platform with him and then-NCI director Frank Rauscher to testify before the Senate's Committee on Labor and Public Welfare to abolish the one-step procedure and to ensure that doctors would inform their patients about alternatives to the Halsted radical mastectomy.[13] Although the white men representing the medical establishment on her panel concurred with her findings, the senators seemed most engaged with Kushner's statements. Her testimony began the hearing and set a precedent both for the subjects discussed and for the perspective that figured most prominently. In that setting the Vietnam War provided a convenient way for Kushner to describe breast cancer to the committee's chair, Senator Edward Kennedy. She characterized the medical issues at stake by referencing the war that preoccupied many people's minds: "To paraphrase the most infamous quote to come out of the war in Vietnam, a mastectomy—too often—destroys a woman's life in order to save it."[14] Her use of a war metaphor forced Kennedy to recognize how the life-threatening controversy was an issue of national urgency. Kushner used—albeit at times uncritically—the cold war rhetoric President Richard Nixon used in his war on cancer when it enabled her to lure a particular audience. In this instance, the language of war situated her as a pivotal member of the army that previously included only white, privileged men in doctor's offices or on Capitol Hill.

Kushner's invocation of the Vietnam War allowed her to engage with counterpublics as well. Introducing a work of poetry about breast cancer twelve years later, she repeated the metaphor she shared with the senators.[15] In so doing she aptly called attention to a war fought inside the body as a parallel to a war fought outside the body on foreign soil. With this metaphor she attracted a wide variety of citizens. Despite its problematic resonances, women with breast cancer often invoke war to describe how they struggle psychically and physically with their disease; but when Kushner invoked Vietnam as an analogy she tapped into Nixon's strategy. However, unlike Nixon, she emphasized the atrocities committed on both fronts and the silence that the government relied on to hide its complicit unethical acts in both wars.

Kushner made it her mission to politicize and publicize the areas of cancer policy that most needed to be changed. She began by revealing the historical reason behind the one-step biopsy and mastectomy in her testimony and in her self-help manual. Placing the institutionalization of the one-step process in context made her commitment to changing the practice understandable: "Instituting the 'two-stage procedure' then became a personal crusade—almost a vendetta, because there is no valid medical reason for combining diagnosis and treatment. The practice is nothing more than a bad habit surgeons acquired as a result of two politico-economic changes that occurred in the United States after World War II" (*Alternatives* 181–182). She accurately identifies these changes. First, the 1946 passage of the Hill-Burton Act gave "local communities federal grants-in-aid to build hospitals all over the country" (*Alternatives* 182). Prior to that, few hospitals even existed in the United States. Moreover, there were very few places where women could have a mastectomy. At that time, doctors extricated women's lumps in their offices and sent them off to a pathologist for diagnosis. If the pathologist confirmed the malignancy of the lump, the woman then traveled to an urban center to have a mastectomy—if she could afford to do so. This routine demonstrated to Kushner that it was merely a myth that a woman needed to have a one-step procedure. Second, the insurance industry further entrenched this one-step practice as it began to refuse payment for surgeries unless they were performed by a hospital surgeon. Such economic and political dilemmas forced biopsies to become inpatient procedures to save women and insurance companies money. The lack of hospital resources, time, and finances forced women to use the reserved hospital time to take care of both the biopsy and the mastectomy at once. With this history Kushner underscored the economic component of this oppressive practice, which inadvertently eliminated women's agency. If the rationale for a one-step biopsy and mastectomy were financial and not medical, then there could be no logical rationale for the practice.

While working to annul the one-step procedure, Crile persuaded Kushner to examine other areas where women with breast cancer lacked alternatives. In Kushner's quest to intervene in this standard surgical practice she learned about the risks of asking a surgeon who performed only Halsted radicals to leave the chest wall intact. In some ways, it was easier and safer for surgeons to take out the entire area than to make a concerted effort to cut around the muscle fibers in the chest. To ask for a different procedure from surgeons would be to risk complications in an otherwise routine procedure because of their inexperience with performing other types of ablation. Crile's medical alternatives needed to be institutionalized in medical school curricula before those surgeries could be widely practiced.

Accordingly, Kushner pushed for another prominent change, in unison with Crile; they demanded that Congress make more surgical options readily and widely available for all women. Although she explained that the location and size of her lump did not make her a candidate for a lumpectomy, she believed women should know about the various kinds of surgeries and have some agency in deciding which one would be best. Just as her research into the one-step procedure yielded an obsolete pretense for an outmoded medical routine, so too did her inquiry into the Halted radical mastectomy: "Although 90 percent of the surgeons in the United States who performed mastectomies, in 1974, did the Halsted radical, I could find no cancer expert—in books or by personal questioning—who thought it was necessary to take out the pectoral muscles" (*Alternatives* 15). She supported this claim by providing readers with a rationale for choosing to have a modified radical mastectomy: "To me, looking as normal as possible minus the breast, having as little scarring as possible, and getting out all of the cancer were the important issues—not the invisible [lymph] nodes. Later, I was to learn about the importance of the nodes in avoiding unnecessary 'frozen shoulder' and lymphedema— swelling of the arm. After reading the literature and telephoning some friends at the National Cancer Institute, I made my choice: a modified radical mastectomy, if my lump turned out to be cancer. My breast and lymph nodes would be removed; the chest muscles controlling my left arm would stay with me" (*Alternatives* 15). The fact that she avoided these debilitating side effects further motivated her to eradicate this deforming surgery.

It was profoundly revolutionary for Kushner to choose her own surgery and then to make her process for doing so public. To that end in a Senate hearing Kushner shared her story about her uphill battle to have a voice in her medical care. In thorough cross-examination, senators uncovered that she visited nineteen surgeons who refused to sign a contract forbidding them to remove her breast at the time of biopsy. She responds to the senators' disbelief by stating: "The 20th surgeon I called thought I was just being a ridiculous 'women's libber,' and he signed the contract."[16] At the height of second-wave feminism, surgeons who found their authority questioned retaliated by not allowing women to control their own lives and bodies. The cross-examination of Kushner on this particular subject continued for a while because the senators appeared quite shocked that no doctor took her request to have a separate biopsy and surgery seriously, despite the fact that her mammograms continued to suggest her lump might be benign. Furthermore, the senators found it even more alarming that there was no medical rationale for the one-step biopsy and mastectomy.

Kushner contested institutionalized practices to get the type of doctor she wanted, the kind of surgery she chose, and the two-stage operation she demanded. But when she received the news that her pathology report diagnosed her lump as malignant, her surgeon described his recommendation without naming it—a Halsted radical mastectomy—and even though she had researched breast cancer treatments extensively, she came close to acquiescing. Indeed, the description caught her by surprise: "I was so terrified by the surgeon's quiet description of the Halsted he proposed to do that it never occurred to me to ask if someone at Sloan-Kettering would do a modified radical mastectomy instead. In my panicky state, I assumed it was standard hospital policy to do Halsteds, not a matter of a surgeon's personal preference" (*Alternatives* 20). Her confession reminded readers that although she was an expert, she too fell prey to the institutional powers of her doctor. Her unconscious inclination makes evident that having a feminist consciousness does not alleviate the quotidian problems of being a woman. Regardless of how much information she armed herself with, being confronted with the loss of a breast rendered her speechless, and at times complacent, in her doctor's presence.

Kushner reiterated these stories, figures, and sentiments in her congressional testimony. There she relied on an economic model that historicized and contextualized the reasons surgeons favored Halsted's radical surgery even after the NCI released its data proving that extracting the pectoral muscles served no medical purpose: "There is a system called the California Relative Value Scale . . . devised by insurance companies. Depending on the part of the country—when I did the research on this, Manhattan was the highest and Montana was the lowest—each kind of surgery is assigned a certain point value. Each point has a specific dollar value for that geographical location. When I checked, a Halsted radical mastectomy was something like 55 or 60 points and [a] modified mastectomy was worth 30 points, and I guess a lumpectomy would be worth 5. Depending on what each point is worth in dollars in that geographical area, that is the way the fee the doctor is paid is calculated."[17] These facts provided a frame of reference for the politicians listening to her testimony. They also highlighted the economic incentives that kept surgeons from offering women choices and from updating their own practices. It was in the surgeon's interest to perform the surgery with the highest compensation.

In her political work, Kushner relied on different rhetorical maneuvers depending on her audience. When she thought it would be effective, she echoed the rhetorical thrust of a woman's right to choose, which resonated with the then-recent Supreme Court decision of *Roe v. Wade.* On the Senate floor and in her writing she capitalized on the already circulating public debates about choice to intervene in a medical practice that seemed peripheral to the dominant public but urgent to women in various counterpublics. But her willingness to let women choose their treatment had its limitations. For example, when First Lady Nancy Reagan chose to have a mastectomy instead of a lumpectomy, Kushner told the *New York Times* that Reagan's choice set women back ten years, although Kushner also conceded that women must be allowed to make their own choices.[18] Reagan decided to have the mastectomy, interestingly, because of her fear of the radiation treatments that would have been necessary if she had chosen the lumpectomy; her decision dramatically affected some women's surgical choices, as Leopold testifies: "In the six months following that diagnosis, there was a 25 percent reduction in the use of breast-conserving surgery as women opted for the same treatment that Nancy Reagan had chosen. Those making that choice were women who, like their role model, were white and over fifty years old; there was apparently no decrease in the use of lumpectomies among African American women" (*A Darker* 252).

Not surprisingly, Kushner's race and class privilege complicated her relationship to feminism. Despite the advent of groundbreaking women's health publications, Kushner still felt that feminists ignored the subject of breast cancer because it was more taboo than abortion and because they were too young to be concerned with it: "We have got to write off the Gloria Steinems; they are deniers, and even if she got breast cancer, even if she has had breast cancer, she'd keep it hidden, whereas she didn't her abortion."[19] Kushner's information here is flawed: Steinem consistently enacted and embodied the feminist tenet that the personal is political. And, moreover, when she did get breast cancer, she wrote about it and discussed it publicly. Indeed, much of Kushner's quest to ensure that women could make their own choices about their bodies depended on the groundwork laid by primarily white, second-wave feminists.

Participating in the burgeoning women's health movement—even on the sidelines of it—called for inherently feminist analyses and tactics, and yet such a strategy risked alienating the privileged white ladies in the dominant public who also needed to hear Kushner's message. Because her early 1970s audience felt anxious about women's libbers, she eases their worries by resorting to Ford's style of white-glove rhetoric to placate skeptical readers: "I must add here, for women's liberationists who see an evil plot to mutilate women by mastectomy, that I found none— anywhere. There has definitely been male chauvinism—enough to warrant a separate chapter later . . . [but] I have found no surgeons, male or female, who had any doubts that radical mastectomy offered women their best chance to survive breast cancer. This—not male chauvinism— is why mastectomies were recommended by almost all surgeons. In 1974, the controversial issues were separating the diagnostic biopsy from mastectomy, what kind of mastectomy should be performed, and who should decide. In my case, the choices were my own" (*Alternatives* 23). This perplexing statement contradicts her earlier claims. She had already stated that she could find no cancer expert who could give any rationale for removing the pectoral muscles, and she also uncovered economic incentives for surgeons based on how much of the body they cut away. Kushner knew these facts, and yet she denied that the systemic forces she was fighting were sexist.

Kushner's seemingly reluctant relationship to feminism can be read as a conflicted statement about the public culture in which she wrote. She wanted to make knowledge about the problems with breast cancer treatment as widespread as possible. In an interview, Kushner attempted to account for this political strategy: "I often joke about having talked to nuns in the morning and lesbians—gays—in the afternoon, and I do and I would talk to the National Rifle Association and the Ku Klux Klan if they asked me; I think that they feel that . . . I'm not politically acceptable."[20] On the one hand, she sometimes embraced a feminist perspective in her writing. On the other hand, she calculated her feminism so she would not alienate anyone who might benefit from her information.

By the way Kushner framed her speaking and writing, she was able to address numerous parallel counterpublics, and at times she engaged directly with the dominant public. Her work in the face of opposing ideological and political forces made her a cultural mediator between counterpublics and the dominant public. Women's lives depended on honest, pragmatic tactics, not simple solutions that merely blamed men or misogyny (as much of the dominant public perceived that feminism's critiques did). Kushner acknowledged the separation between her personal decisions and her later role as an advocate. She believed that her story, combined with the scientific data in her text, would encourage all women to draw their own conclusions about their bodies.

Kushner understood the necessity for a vital flow of information and fought to create legislation that ensured women would have access to it.

One of the bills she worked to introduce in Congress was the Breast Cancer Informed Consent law. Only eighteen state legislatures eventually passed this bill, which would have required doctors to provide "information on treatment, specifically alternatives to radical mastectomy";[21] to obtain consent "from the patient herself *prior* to surgery" and to penalize doctors "for physician noncompliance" (Anglin 1405). Mary Anglin points out that this piece of legislation was "largely symbolic in content, women with breast cancer achieved success in the sense that they were able to use personal testimony to lobby state legislatures and to publicize the issue of breast cancer through the media" (1405).[22] And indeed most of these requirements were put into practice in most places within the next decade merely by using the media to highlight the personal narratives of women like Kushner. In this respect, her work as a writer and activist eventually led to new relationships and better communication between doctors and patients, as Wendy Schain points out: "Rose Kushner . . . contributed immeasurably to the changes that have taken place in breast cancer management" (933).

Although her books are out of print and outdated, Kushner's legacy remains vital because she tirelessly and publicly questioned the medical treatments for breast cancer patients in the 1970s and 1980s. Her writings and her testimony before Congress brought about concrete results;[23] specifically, women eventually won the right to a two-stage procedure. And, largely because of the public consciousness raised by Kushner, in the last edition of her book she reported that Halsted radical mastectomies were almost obsolete.[24] Kushner's activism embodied the way women actively fought to secure some agency in their surgical treatment. Like most breast cancer patients regardless of race, class, or sexuality, she worried about scars, complications, and disfigurement. That she made a choice to minimize these concerns for herself and for other women remains extraordinary.

ACTIVIST MEMORIALIZING

To a certain extent Rose Kushner never gained the same access to the public sphere that Betty Ford will always have. But the cultural, political, and public groundwork Kushner laid for herself and for other women can be felt even now, more than a decade after her death in January 1990. She facilitated numerous changes for patient's rights through her Breast Cancer Advisory Center, which became one of the first advocacy organizations for women with breast cancer. For instance, on a public level, in 1974 she won a landmark lawsuit against the U.S. Department of Health and Human Services and the Food and Drug Administration requiring manufacturers of birth-control pills to place a label on their products warning women with breast cancer to avoid using pills as a method of contraception. On a private level, she volunteered her support to women faced with breast cancer: "Her counseling efforts [were] so well known that the post office routinely deliver[ed] to her letters addressed 'Mrs. Breast Cancer, Kensington, Maryland'" (Johnson 160). She also cofounded the first national breast cancer advocacy and fundraising group in the country, the National Alliance of Breast Cancer Organizations, and continued her appointed work with the NCI, the ACS, and the Presidential National Cancer Advisory Board. When she died, she left behind her last lobbying project: for state and federal legislation to offer Medicare and Medicaid coverage for mammography, as well as to allocate more research dollars to breast cancer. This work was dynamic and pioneering. She invaded the most public, entrenched grounds of the exclusive white, male bureaucracy: the Senate and the NCI. And her efforts demonstrate the powerful ways in which one woman writing about her breast cancer can effect changes in public policy and medical practices.[25]

As a testament to the ways that Kushner irrevocably altered the medical landscape, a public memorial pays tribute to her activism and writing. A traveling photographic show entitled "The Face of Breast Cancer" commemorates a fairly diverse group of eighty-four women representing every state. The exhibit features Rose Kushner on the right-hand side of one panel (Figure 4). Although she is not the focus of the exhibit, the profile head shot of her smiling face represents her tireless positive energy. These photographs travel the country but also get displayed in the rotunda of the Russell Senate Office Building during the National Breast Cancer Coalition's (NBCC) annual lobby day. Kushner's photograph and the biographical essay placed next to it infuse this dominant public space with a significant feminist presence by politicizing the exhibit's intended call to action. With this show, the NBCC seeks to humanize the statistics of breast cancer and to highlight the epidemic by asking passersby to see the faces of the forty-six thousand women who die of breast cancer each year.

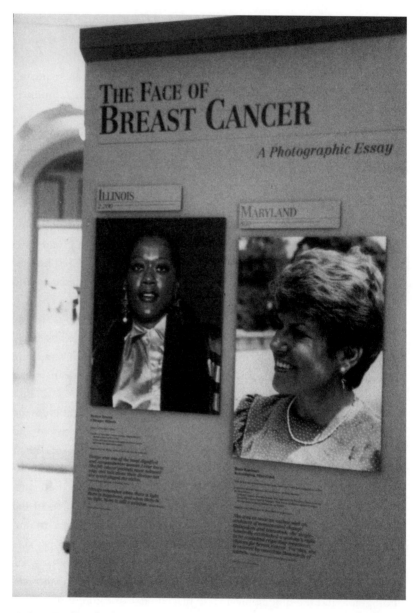

4. Rose Kushner (right) in the "Face of Breast Cancer" exhibit. NBCC The Face of Breast Cancer Exhibit, May 1997.

This public memorial resonates with other representations of disease in public culture. Like the Names Project AIDS Memorial Quilt, the NBCC's photographic exhibit presents a public communal space where grieving merges with a pedagogical and political moment. As an artistic and political text, the memorial explicitly calls attention to the epidemic itself. And it also resonates with memorials that commemorate those who served and died in the armed forces. The difference with this memorial, however, is that it does not represent solely the loss of life; rather, it asks viewers to remember that these women helped to end silences within the medical and political spheres. Like the memorial in Washington, D.C., honoring soldiers killed in Vietnam, such public art, argues literary critic Carole Blair, performs two crucial tasks: "First, [the Vietnam Memorial] announced that those who had served their country were worthy of memory, despite the embarrassing military outcome. Second, it marked a place for the veterans and survivors of the dead (as well as others) to come together and form a community of recognition, grieving, healing, and activism that had been all but missing from the public sphere" (34). I would argue that the "Face of Breast Cancer" exhibit, honoring women who died from cancer, works similarly. It opens up and reminds us of a time when breast cancer was shrouded in secrecy. This artistic monument was created by a group of feminist cancer activists, and their work functions as a grieving and healing site as well as a place to commune and plan the next direct action or legislative strategy to procure increased funding for breast cancer research. Memorializing the work of these women who did not survive breast cancer reminds activists of those whom their work for legislative changes honors.

Kushner created texts that intervened in and contested previous oversights in breast cancer treatment. To a certain extent, Ford's white-glove rhetoric influenced her texts by provoking Kushner to bear witness to breast cancer, raise women's consciousness, and change the political and medical landscape in the process. But one aspect of Ford's and Kushner's consciousness-raising efforts that remains unfinished in a pronounced manner is a nuanced and sustained engagement with the ways that race, sexuality, and socioeconomic class affect women's interactions with—or lack of action in—the medical sphere. As many critiques of the women's liberation movement articulate, mainstream white women's feminism often elides the concerns of women of color, poor women, and lesbians. The hypervisibility of white, middle-class women inadvertently and at times overtly erased or silenced women of color, lesbians, and poor women in ways that contribute to tangible inequities in medical practices and mortality rates. It took one woman who straddled all these categories to bring these overlapping concerns into the public sphere. That woman was Audre Lorde.

CHAPTER 4

Toward Truth and Reconciliation

AUDRE LORDE'S REVISION OF
BREAST CANCER NARRATIVES

ROSE KUSHNER tackled the medical establishment by taking a two-pronged approach in Congress and in the halls of the National Cancer Institute (NCI); in doing so, she imagined that her choices would be choices that all women would necessarily embrace. The notion that saving the breast at all costs would not be a priority for every woman never seemed to occur to her. Too, when she spoke or wrote about breast cancer, her ethnicity and sexuality were rendered invisible to her audience; as a privileged, white, Jewish, heterosexual woman she was not conscious of the ways in which her body was racially marked and how that factored into the normalizing gaze of the dominant public. Like many white, Western feminists during the women's liberation movement, she was concerned primarily with issues she believed to be universal: namely, changing U.S./Western medical practices to allow all women a voice in shaping them. Like Betty Ford, Kushner did not have a heightened consciousness about the nuanced ways in which breast cancer affected poor women, women of color, and lesbians. She certainly made substantial changes in ways that enact Audre Lorde's call to transforming silence into language and action, but these changes were still focused primarily on white, heterosexual women. Specific differences among women—race, class, sexuality, nationality—remained absent from medical and governmental discourse about breast cancer, and medical studies of mortality and incidence rates had yet to incorporate these vital epidemiological data.

This chapter describes how Audre Lorde, someone who carried the burden of multiple identities—black, lesbian, feminist, mother, "warrior poet"—broke the silence within feminist public spheres about the ways in which compulsory white heteronormativity and femininity negatively affect the emotional and physical healing process for many women. Voicing concerns that had previously been silenced, she also critiqued the generally unquestioned practices of U.S./Western medicine and the role of the environment in increasing cancer incidence rates.

To be sure, Lorde had done her homework: she had read Kushner as well as Samuel Epstein, both of whom she cites in her journals. Their political work, Kushner as a breast cancer survivor and Epstein as a medical doctor and environmental lobbyist, made Lorde's experiences with the medical establishment more tolerable than they might otherwise have been. Because of their efforts Lorde knew she had choices about her treatment, and she learned that environmental connections to the disease had not yet been studied in a serious way. Kushner's book *Breast Cancer* alerted Lorde to the option of a two-stage operation separating the biopsy from the surgery. Although a feminist like Lorde might have asserted her voice in the medical process in any case, Kushner's research documenting that there were no sound medical reasons for a one-step procedure helped Lorde navigate Beth Israel Hospital in New York City.

However, for the most part, unlike the case for the women highlighted in previous chapters, I cannot trace a direct link between Lorde's work and concrete changes made in medical and public policy regarding breast cancer or among breast cancer patients themselves. Like Rachel Carson, Ford, and Kushner, Lorde's purpose in writing an autobiographical text was not solely to aid her own healing process. Rather, she published *The Cancer Journals* and later *A Burst of Light* with the intention that other cancer survivors, women, and doctors would read her work.[1] And indeed they have—with *The Cancer Journals* being her most popular and best-selling work.[2] And although I cannot credit her with changes doctors may have made in the way they treat their patients or the empowerment breast cancer patients may have experienced with respect to their bodies, her narrative played a part in shaping the way that many African American women and lesbians think about their bodies during and after breast cancer. I believe that Lorde's texts have had a tremendous impact on the rethinking of a woman's postmastectomy body; they have challenged standard Western medical practices, questioned the role of the environment in cancer causation, and created a consciousness about the absence of race, class, and sexuality in medical discourse. Although it remains outside the scope of this project to trace specific audience reception of her books, in the final section of this chapter I allude to the possibility that since the publication of her manuscripts in the 1980s her work has transformed patients, activists, doctors, and writers.

In this chapter I examine what Lorde did best: melding poetic language and narrative form in order to effectively articulate her class-conscious, global, queer, feminist, and antiracist politics. In the process of excavating the genre of autobiography, Lorde carved out a space for other narratives to emerge after hers in various feminist counterpublic spheres. Ultimately, I argue, Lorde transformed a generation of feminists and activists who created innovative direct-action organizations and shaped public policy in ways that continue the work she laid out in her books.

Specifically, in *The Cancer Journals* Lorde reconceived the formal structure of autobiography by subverting reader's expectations, although the genre is ascribed to women and has historically been utilized by African Americans and women as a consciousness-raising tool. Her narrative calls attention to the various issues that arise for women with breast cancer depending on their identities as feminists, African Americans, poor, or lesbians. By the time she elaborated her autobiographical narrative in *A Burst of Light* she had extended her consciousness-raising project to interrogate standardized Western medical treatments for cancer, while also posing questions that led readers to consider the environmental links to breast cancer. Lorde's narrative structure, although different in *A Burst of Light and The Cancer Journals*, supports her arguments by not being a traditional chronological, linear recounting of or reflection on her life experiences.

In *The Cancer Journals* Lorde revises the typical autobiographical narrative form by commencing with a speech she gave at a 1977 Modern Language Association (MLA) meeting; the initial subject of the speech is Winnie Mandela and South African apartheid. Opening her journal with models for resistance that are familiar to many of her readers, she imagines the silence surrounding apartheid in dominant discourse within a variety of global public spheres as analogous to the silence about breast cancer. In some ways one becomes a metaphor for the other; both are systemic, spatial, and forms of disease—and, most important, both can be challenged.[3] In this speech she famously urged listeners to use the power of language and to reclaim "that language which has been made to work against us. In the transformation of silence into language and action, it is vitally necessary for each one of us to establish or examine her function in that transformation, and to recognize her role as vital within that transformation" (*Cancer* 21). Lorde lived by those words.

Taking my cue from her imperative, I explore the ways in which Lorde's writing transformed silence into language and action by building on the momentum begun by women who publicly discussed other aspects of breast cancer before her. To explore the possibility of her contribution to altering the course of standard medical procedures and patient responses to those practices, I engage with the aspect of Lorde's cancer writing that readers may be most familiar with: her challenge to heteronormative standards of beauty that enforced the use of prosthetic breasts to conceal and censor the postmastectomy body. She created a paradigm shift that raised the consciousness of medical professionals and breast cancer survivors alike about the ways in which concealing one's body inhibits healing one's body. Her analysis of these hegemonic practices signaled the theme that unifies the entire corpus of her work: the necessity of giving voice to the silenced.

One of the suppressed subjects that she made visible was the effect of race, class, and sexuality on women who are encountering the medical sphere. To a certain extent, the narrative and political trajectory that she followed extends back to slave narratives in which black women bore witness to the lack of control they had over their bodies on a number of levels. For enslaved women, and for Lorde, writing was a part of surviving. In one sense Lorde connected herself to that legacy by grounding her texts in an autobiographical mode and by linking breast cancer to a modern version of colonialism as evidenced in South African apartheid. In another sense, the urgency of apartheid mirrors the urgency of her cancer when it metastasized to her liver and thereby provided a powerful lesson in the myriad ways that silence equals pain, trauma, and death. Using her writing as a tool for survival, Lorde illustrated with her body and her voice the necessity of testifying to the oppressive ways in which women of the African diaspora have not controlled their own bodies.

In this chapter I also trace the ways in which liver metastasis pushed Lorde to reflect on standard Western beliefs about cancer treatment and causation and the limitations within those paradigms for controlling one's own body. In *A Burst of Light* she employs a diary format to chronicle her experience with holistic treatment in Germany and Switzerland as well as her organizing against apartheid with African women and women of the African diaspora. A change in her physical surroundings and medical treatment produced amended theories about the interconnectedness of racism, poverty, cancer, and the environment; she alludes to this growing concern and her struggles with it: "At the poetry reading in Zurich this weekend, I found it so much easier to discuss racism than to talk about *The Cancer Journals*. Chemical plants between Zurich and Basel have been implicated in a definite rise in breast cancer in this region, and women wanted to discuss this" (*Burst* 60). With this text, then, Lorde shifted the debate from inside women's bodies to outside their bodies—a rhetorical move that enabled her simultaneously to lift the blame from women and to place it on the polluting environmental corporations, some of which Carson first called attention to fifteen years earlier. Lorde ended her breast cancer writing on this note, and in so doing she reiterated and built on the struggle of African Americans to control their bodies and their environment.

Transformation(s)

Two years before Lorde's death in 1990, *Callaloo* editor Charles Rowell interviewed her, asking her specifically about how she hoped readers of her poetry would respond to it. Her answer to that question provides significant insight into Lorde's intentions as a writer. She replied, "I want my poems—I want all of my work—to engage, and to empower people to speak, to strengthen themselves into who they most want and need to be and then to act, to do what needs to be done. In other words, learn to use themselves in the service of what they believe" (62). Art and politics are inseparable for Lorde, as she explained to Rowell: "We are living in a sick society, and any art which does not serve change—i.e., does not speak the truth—is beside the point" (61). For people who know Lorde's writing and political work, these concepts may seem familiar. But her theory about the use value of literature bears repeating. Lorde believed that art could be the catalyst for progressive social change. To that end, she did not differentiate between speaking with one's words or with one's body. The political foundation of her life's work tied the poetry she created to the body that produced it. And indeed with her first volume of narrative prose, *The Cancer Journals,* Lorde made these links explicit.

The way Lorde melds words and images together on a page of poems to give voice to a truth does not differ tremendously from the way she constructs her prose. The inventiveness and playfulness with which she crafts her autobiographical/essay writing is equally, deliberately impassioned. From the first chapter of *The Cancer Journals* readers confront the fact that they are not reading an ordinary journal, memoir, autobiography, or diary, as the title promises. Although her introduction certainly alerts readers to her unusual form, the first chapter supports her disruption of generic form. Opening the volume with the speech she delivered on Mandela during the lesbian and literature panel at the MLA meeting may at first seem unrelated to the title of the book and that of the panel. She introduces the work of Mandela to her audience through a poem Lorde wrote about Mandela's exile and struggle against apartheid in South Africa. The refrain in the poem—"our uses have become / more important than our silence"—combines broader themes calling listeners to action (*Cancer* 17).[4] In a call-and-response style of delivery, Lorde builds on the call that the title of her talk—"The Transformation of Silence into Language and Action"—alludes to. The concept that silence equals death—and that a vocal call to action can be a method of survival—leads her to the crescendo, in which she utters her most oft-repeated refrain—"My silences had not protected me. Your silence will not protect you"—to publicly disclose her then-recent breast cancer diagnosis (*Cancer* 18). For Lorde it does not matter what the silence is; the concern is that there is a silence at all.

Like most of her work Lorde's feminist mantra—which rings in concert with the work of white feminist writers like Tillie Olsen and Adrienne Rich—is fundamentally about using language as a call to action: "Because I am woman, because I am black, because I am lesbian, because I am myself, a black woman warrior poet doing my work, [I] come to ask you, are you doing yours?" (*Cancer* 19). Her question is not rhetorical. Rather, it indicates Lorde's dialogic style. She made her call, and she seeks a real response from the audience. There is an urgency to gathering a critical mass to overthrow the Afrikaner regime. Likewise, there is an urgency she feels in her body because cancer forces her to question her own mortality. Despite the implicit danger inherent in putting one's words or body on the line, Lorde does not have a choice. Her politics demand that she challenge the deadly silences that most often affect people of color, women, poor people, and queer people. Given that she was addressing a room full of writers and teachers, it is significant that she asked them to consider the power of the words that one reads, writes, and teaches, for one method of combating these silences and making survival possible is linking language to action.

The words that emanated from Lorde's mouth were firmly rooted in her body—that is, she spoke simultaneously from and of her body. It was imperative for her to use her voice and body to speak about black women's survival in the broadest possible sense because when she spoke or wrote, she did so, consciously, on behalf of so many women of the African diaspora who could not, did not. Elizabeth Alexander makes this case convincingly and clearly: "Lorde maps the new terrain of what over 100 years ago Linda Brent [*Incidents in the Life of a Slave Girl Written by Herself (Harriet Jacobs)*] had to whisper and withhold from her readers: all that a corporeal history embodies. The link between Lorde and Brent is crucial: for both, the issue is control over one's own body and the power to see the voice as a literal functioning *member* of the corpus, an organ that works and must be self-tended" ("Coming" 713). Indeed, Alexander's connection between *Incidents in the Life of a Slave Girl* and *The Cancer Journals* is insightful. It informs Lorde's unique response to breast cancer by connecting silences in her bodily context with silences in the context of Mandela's embodied suffering. This relationship between racist political repression and cancer is not an empty metaphorical gesture. Rather, the fact and urgency of apartheid and the systemic forms of racism, sexism, homophobia, and classism in the United States ultimately compelled Lorde to push public debates toward discussions of cancer as a systemic disease stemming from environmental contaminants. Lorde spoke and wrote through all these complex, entangled subjects because they were inscribed in and on her body. Linda Brent/Harriet Jacobs had to whisper from behind the veil of a pseudonym so that Lorde could scream—shout if necessary—on behalf of herself and other women of the African diaspora.

The historical weight of black women like Brent/Jacobs and the present pressure of African women like Mandela compelled Lorde to write with her body, to bear witness as a means for taking control of her body. Breaking up the chronological linearity of her narrative, she begins the second section of her memoir with a 1978 diary entry. Interspersed between these entries are her reflections on those narratives, each one interrupting and amplifying the other in much the same way that cancer seemed to have affected her life. In her writing dated October 5, 1978, she demonstrates the embodied process of writing: "The act of writing seems impossible to me sometimes, the space of time for the words to form or be written is long enough for the situation to totally alter, leaving you liar or at search once again for the truth. What seems impossible is made real/tangible by the physical form of my brown arm moving across the page; not that my arm cannot do it, but that something holds it away" (*Cancer* 53). Writing and being are inseparable. Each one gives way to the other. It was important for her to write through these painful gaps in her thoughts because of its use value for those who did not, could not write with their bodies. Thus, writing through the body had the potential to end silences not only for her but for those who would read her words. Finding truth in her writing was as necessary as revealing the truth of her body—her new one-breasted body—especially given a historical context in which black women had not had the power to decide or determine how others read or treated their bodies; Lorde knew that owning and honoring her new body could be of use to herself and to others.

Perhaps this impetus to place one's body and voice on the line on behalf of other black, lesbian, or feminist women compelled Lorde to create more of a polemic than a journal. If the MLA speech that opens her book alerts readers to the ways in which Lorde disrupts narrative form, the politics of her prose and of her body mimic that gesture. Publicly demonstrating that she intervened in her breast cancer treatment by making choices to refuse reconstruction, prosthesis, radiation, and chemotherapy indicated yet another way in which Lorde interrupted and called attention to cycles of control and oppression over bodies belonging to brown-skinned, lesbian, poor women.[5] Indeed, Lorde embraced a body that the dominant public treats as distorted, disabled, disfigured. I would locate this corporeal, narrative trend in the same impulse that motivated Brent/Jacobs. Nellie McKay defines such a gesture as a form of empowerment: "The narratives of Brent and others of her time illustrate that black survival (their own and that of others) not the quest to recuperate lost selves, motivated these women's active subversion of black victimization. They turned to their own resources and discovered a power within their powerlessness that enabled them to resist the devastating impact of white power over the black self" (100).

I would not argue that the process of surviving breast cancer was the same as the process of escaping and surviving slavery. I do want to suggest, however, that these histories and narratives of black women's bodies are deeply intertwined. Lorde knew where this power resides and how to access it even though/even when, in her journal, she grappled with gradations of suffering, pain, grief, and despair. But giving voice to her pain explicitly was precisely what gave her and her readers power. Therefore, one of the historical elements she traces through this journal is the uphill battle of black women to survive historically in the United States. Lorde suggests, "To survive in the mouth of this dragon we call america, we have had to learn this first and most vital lesson—that we were never meant to survive" (*Cancer* 20). The we, of course, refers to African Americans and to the legacy of slavery. Facing her mortality seemed to bridge this historical gap and the political/social context of survival for African American women. Lorde found herself facing off against various forces in the medical sphere, an indication that remnants of McKay's formulation about empowering black women had currents running through the white, heterosexual, male, Western paradigm that dominated the medical establishment Lorde found herself in the thick of.

Lorde's first autobiographical prose writing is most often remembered for its resistance to the dominant and largely unquestioned practices within the medical arena. Clearly, even the strides that Kushner made—even when she reached out to feminists, lesbians, or African Americans—did not meet the needs of a defiantly one-breasted, black lesbian, feminist, mother, warrior poet. Neither Kushner nor Ford had to confront the multiple contexts that Lorde had to, contexts in which her identity was erased or amplified. And there was no support system in place in African American communities.[6] Lorde recalls when a well-intentioned, middle-aged, white woman with breast cancer visited Lorde after her mastectomy on behalf of the Reach for Recovery Program of the American Cancer Society: (ACS). "Her message was, you are just as good as you were before because you can look exactly the same. Lambswool now, then a good prosthesis as soon as possible, and nobody'll ever know the difference. But what she said was, '*You'll* never know the difference,' and she lost me right there, because I knew sure as hell *I'd* know the difference" (*Cancer* 42). At this moment Lorde wonders where all the black lesbian feminists with breast cancer are. Her issues and concerns were not surviving in the heterosexual dating pool, as might have been the case for this woman. Rather she wanted to heal, and she wanted to do so in the company of women with whom she shared a common language. Lorde did not care whether she would find a husband. She wanted to know what it would be like when three breasts brushed against each other rather than four when she made love with her partner, Frances Clayton.

Indeed, the notion that one can ignore the reality of the loss of one's breast by the use of compulsory, heteronormative prosthetic devices spoke to Lorde of larger concerns. Such a masquerade was impossible for her as a woman of the African diaspora. She could not conceal the fact of her flesh and the ways it prohibited her from blending in. As she eloquently elaborates, "I am personally affronted by the message that I am only acceptable if I look 'right' or 'normal,' where those norms have nothing to do with my own perceptions of who I am. Where 'normal' means the 'right' color, shape, size, or number of breasts, a woman's perception of her own body and the strengths that come from that perception are discouraged, trivialized, and ignored" (*Cancer* 66). Some might read the surface of Lorde's words as addressing only the cosmetic aspects of one's body and the various ways one perceives herself and the way others perceive her. But, in fact, her critical distance from prostheses enabled women to approach their bodies in a way that contributed to their healing process. The key for Lorde was that she believed a woman should have time and space "to accept her new body" first before placing a puff of lamb's wool or a silicone device into her bra (*Cancer* 65). The imperative for her to encourage women to accept the body they have been presented with came from her experience living in a racist, homophobic, misogynist world. She understood that "certain other people feel better with that lump stuck into my bra, because they do not have to deal with me nor themselves in terms of mortality nor in terms of difference" (*Cancer* 65). Therefore, the process of accepting the terrain of her new torso was embedded within the ways in which she embraced all the complex facets of her identity and of the ways in which her body was visibly marked as different.

In the introduction to *The Cancer Journals*, Lorde makes it quite clear that she does not object to women who attempt to make their postmastectomy bodies resemble their former physical exterior. As a feminist she saw making choices about one's body as fundamentally a part of her politics. For those who may have misread her previously, she clarifies her argument: "It is not my intention to judge the woman who has chosen the path of prosthesis, of silence and invisibility, the woman who wishes to be 'the same as before.' She has survived on another kind of courage, and she is not alone. Each of us struggles daily with the pressures of conformity and the loneliness of difference from which those choices seem to offer escape" (*Cancer* 8).[7] As someone amply aware of the oppressive, institutional forces at work trying to control women's bodies, Lorde did not make blanket statements arguing that all women must not wear prostheses. That nurses silenced her body after her modified radical mastectomy by forcing her to wear a prosthesis was yet another episode in a long history of white, heteronormative institutions controlling black women's bodies. It was an attempt to determine and define her experience, her body, her being.

The rush to cover up the scar, the pain, the new and different body created a compulsory heteronormative climate that was antithetical to Lorde's intuitive method of healing. In some ways this oppressive climate was yet another incarnation of a lack of consciousness on the part of nurses and other healthcare workers whose aim was certainly to comfort and heal their cancer patients. Each barrier that women with breast cancer encountered in the 1960s and 1970s that limited their agency within the medical process was generally invisible. Until a woman with cancer put a name to it or put it in writing, women had limited access to medical information and the choices available to them. The burden was on the woman who was trying to recover; the effect was that she often found herself doing battle with the cancer and with the medical system. Although Kushner's exhaustive research facilitated Lorde's navigation of surgical options, it did not address needs particularized to women's race, sexuality, or class. Therefore, when Lorde called attention to the occasions on which she encountered medical professionals who believed that "'it's bad for the morale of the office'" to go to a doctor's appointment without wearing the lamb's wool puff, she named an unspoken silence (*Cancer* 60). Incredibly it is as if Lorde was the only patient in the office—indeed in any office at the time—who noticed the irony in her situation: "Every woman there either had a breast removed, might have to have a breast removed, or was afraid of having to have a breast removed. And every woman there could have used a reminder that having one breast did not mean her life was over, nor that she was less a woman, nor that she was condemned to the use of a placebo in order to feel good about the way she looked" (*Cancer* 61). It struck Lorde as particularly odd that in the supposed safety of the surgeon's office women were confronted with a compelling need to mask the "changed landscape" of their bodies (*Cancer* 61).

This compulsory hiding of one's removed breast led Lorde to compare this phenomenon to the situation of then–Foreign Minister Moshe Dayan of Israel, who "stands up in front of parliament or on TV with an eyepatch over his empty eyesocket, [and] nobody tells him to go get a glass eye, or that he is bad for the morale of the office. . . . If you have trouble dealing with Moshe Dayan's empty eye socket, everyone recognizes that it is your problem to solve, not his" (*Cancer* 61). Lorde questioned the practice of covering up bodies with missing parts and described the way racism, misogyny, and homophobia collide when bodies visibly challenge normative standards of being, of beauty. Let me be clear: I do not mean that the nurses suggesting to Lorde that she wear a prosthesis or forcing her to do so did so consciously. Rather, the fact that an otherwise able-bodied, white, heterosexual, male head of state did not find his body even up for discussion summoned this compelling analogy. Moreover, the fact that it was Dayan's eye that had been removed alludes to the theme of in/visibility, which connects all Lorde's writing and politics. Here too the irony was not lost on Lorde.

What Lorde was getting at in her analysis of prostheses is the way in which women with breast cancer are kept apart from one another. Whether deliberate or not, silencing their bodies with an imitative device suppresses their voices as well. Thus, when Lorde searched for other lesbians or African American women to talk to about her surgery and healing process, she found it a rather daunting prospect. And in fact when Lorde met a member of her extended family who had survived breast cancer for ten years, they squashed another silence by speaking about the particularities of mastectomy scars on African American women's bodies. Li'l Sister, her brother-in-law's younger sister, comforted Lorde, even though they had not known each other previously. Lorde says, "Li'l Sister and I were deeply and busily engaged in discussing our surgeries, including pre- and post-mastectomy experiences. We compared notes on nurses, exercises, and whether or not cocoa-butter retarded black women's tendencies to keloid, the process by which excess scar tissue is formed to ward off infection" (*Cancer* 51). Kushner's book did not explain these aspects of the postsurgical experience, and the staff at Beth Israel could not help Lorde with them. Speaking a common, embodied language was dependent on not tidily covering up unpleasant or uncomfortable silences. For Lorde her body, voice, and mind were intertwined; and to function as if they were not would have been to inhibit her recovery. She explains what it feels like to be silenced: "The emphasis upon wearing a prosthesis is a way of avoiding having women come to terms with their own pain and loss, and thereby, with their own strength" (*Cancer* 49).

The critique Lorde launched in this slim volume was not a simplistic, feminist statement about the oppressive nature of prosthetic devices. Instead, she forwarded an argument that challenged the Western medical system, which separated the mind from the body throughout the healing process. The growing power of antiapartheid activists working together was yet another piece of evidence that voice and visibility equal power, truth, and healing.

A polemic essay constitutes the final chapter of her journal; in it Lorde crystallizes her argument in the most crucial way: "If we are to translate the silence surrounding breast cancer into language and action against this scourge, then the first step is that women with mastectomies must become visible to each other. For silence and invisibility go hand in hand with powerlessness. By accepting the mask of prosthesis, one-breasted women proclaim ourselves as insufficients dependent upon pretense. We reinforce our own isolation and invisibility from each other, as well as the false complacency of a society which would rather not face the results of its own insanities" (*Cancer* 62–63). To a certain extent Kushner was also aware of the need for women with breast cancer to be connected to one another, although in a different sense. Neither woman wanted to see other women with breast cancer separated from one another. Both used their writing to empower other writers, women, and activists and to give them some tools for making choices about how their bodies could be treated.

Being cognitively and consciously in touch with her body led Lorde to expand and elaborate many of the issues developed in *The Cancer Journals* in *A Burst of Light*. Indeed, the title refers to "inescapable knowledge, in the bone of my own physical limitation. Metabolized and integrated into the fabric of my days, that knowledge makes the particulars of what is coming seem less important" (*Burst* 121). Cancer, by this writing, had become integrated into Lorde's identity. The narrative form here and its subject take author and reader alike on a slightly more urgent journey. In contradistinction to *The Cancer Journals* Lorde's last volume of prose, published eight years later, appears at first glance to be an essay collection more like *Sister Outsider*. There is no claim that this book is a "journal." Indeed, Lorde calls it an "essay" in the acknowledgments and on the book jacket. Moreover, she makes no unifying claims about the materials between the covers. Instead, contained in this slim volume are two pamphlets previously published by Kitchen Table: Women of Color Press: "I Am Your Sister: Black Women Organizing across Sexualities" and "Apartheid U.S.A." Two other articles focus on lesbian parenting and sadomasochism. But the book closes with the essay Lorde calls "A Burst of Light: Living with Cancer." Although she grounds this piece in a particular genre—and it has an introduction and an epilogue contained within it—the narrative reads most closely like a diary or a journal. In fact, this essay is much more of a journal about cancer than *The Cancer Journals*, although this fact might be lost on women with cancer otherwise unfamiliar with Lorde's work.

Thematically speaking, this essay resembles *The Cancer Journals* in important ways. Just as the various facets of Lorde's identities cannot be separated, her political work and poetic writing cannot be broken down into the various concerns that permeate her texts. Thus, while "A Burst of Light" chronicles Lorde's metastasis to the liver six years after her mastectomy, much of this narrative is also about her organizing work on behalf of women living under apartheid. Reading these two volumes together, in fact, vibrantly illustrates what it means to transform silence into language and action. Where she writes a poem on behalf of Mandela in the first book, in the second book she teaches her readers how to engage in political organizing on behalf of South African women. Much as in her first prose journal, here too she weaves in recursive interrupting sequences of reflection and explanation about various moments described in the diary entries. If Lorde's form seems more conventional than usual in this semisequel, her content is anything but. This book is one of the first to lay out and document different medical approaches to cancer—approaches used in Europe and in the United States, homeopathic treatments and traditional treatments. And, all of this explication remains firmly ensconced within her larger projects of fighting for black women's self-determination and survival.

SILENCE

For Lorde in the late 1970s and 1980s two items on her agenda were of equal importance and were seemingly insurmountable. One was South African apartheid, and the other was her diagnosis and metastasis of breast cancer. She lays out this agenda and its imperative explicitly: "Battling racism and battling heterosexism and battling apartheid share the same urgency inside me as battling cancer" (*Burst* 116). Given Lorde's extraordinary political commitment and vision, it is likely that at some point she would have seen the connection between systemic disease and its effect on black, queer, and poor women's health and the systemic oppression she experienced and witnessed in a variety of contexts. But the word *urgent* appears here and elsewhere in her writing with increasing frequency once she is diagnosed with breast cancer and is faced with her own mortality. Important in this iteration too is the location not merely of the cancer, which obviously is inside her body, but also of the isms (racism, heterosexism). Thus, the topographic space of her body and its boundaries inside and outside can be thought of as blurred. By empathizing with women who lived under the apartheid regime, she internalized their pain as a way to imagine literary and political solutions to resisting and dismantling it.

Rather than positing that Lorde's body—or any body for that matter—holds some essential nature, I see her text as examining and utilizing the movement and energy and knowledge that travels within her body. Zillah Eisenstein articulates how this process worked for her as she thought through the corporeal, political meanings of her breast cancer: "I do not see the female body as having a natural essence or some kind of true meaning. Rather, it is always embroiled with powerful cultural narratives and their psychic meanings. Bodies are intellectually challenging and environmentally porous. The borders are not simple or unchanging, and, therefore, neither are we" (39). Applied to Lorde's writing, her body takes in the political struggles that affect her. The dominant cultural narratives of her past and present are a part of her flesh. Power is embedded within her, and she uses that power to rewrite the dominant narratives that erase or elide cultural difference in ways that inflict various forms of violence.

Juxtaposing parallel battles not only facilitates Lorde's political organizing but also becomes a tool she uses in her healing process. Meaning, power, and her usefulness as a poet merge in the shadow of metastasis and mortality. As Lorde explains, "I spend time every day meditating upon my physical self in battle, visualizing the actual war going on inside my body. As I move through the other parts of each day, that battle often merges with particular external campaigns, both political and personal. The devasations of apartheid in South Africa and racial murder in Howard Beach feel as critical to me as cancer" (*Burst* 125). This amplification of the parallels she draws between the oppressions described above demonstrates the fluid motion of energy from external to internal, personal to political, until all these waged wars blend together within the meditation and visualization process. The truth that comes out is that brown bodies are on the line regardless of context. She made this connection clear in *The Cancer Journals* when she documented the then-current statistics about the disproportionate rates at which black and poor women acquire and die from breast cancer. "As women, we cannot afford to look the other way, nor to consider the incidence of breast cancer as a private nor secret personal problem. It is no secret that breast cancer is on the increase among women in America. According to the American Cancer Society's own statistics on breast cancer survival, of the women stricken, only 50% are still alive after three years. This figure drops 30% if you are poor, or Black or in any other way part of the underside of this society" (*Cancer* 63). This statistical reality tints the lens through which Lorde examined cancer. In so doing she uncovered a silence that at the time had not even registered on the radar screen of most medical researchers or professionals.

One can see from a Medline search that in the 1970s only 81 medical studies on breast cancer out of a total of 5,704 even mentioned race as a category to be taken into consideration in research. Linking race and breast cancer or thinking comprehensively about that relationship did not become substantive and commonplace until the mid-1990s. It is possible that Lorde's writing helped to push the cultural and political climate of cancer study in this direction. And, in fact, sales of *The Cancer Journals* to medical schools have increased since the early 1990s as curriculum changes have paved the way for courses on patients' perspectives and rights.[8] Moreover, Lorde made it clear that this was not merely a genetic issue. She never argued that black women or poor women had defective genes. Rather, she maintained that these statistics reflected an increase because oppressive forces ignored brown-skinned and poor citizens in a segregated nation. Living conditions for poor African Americans may not have been the same as for South African blacks or coloureds, but as Lorde suggests in much of her prose, limited power, mobility, and resources give way to toxic environments.

By seamlessly sealing together previously disparate subjects under the rubric of silence, Lorde effectively shifts how we think about breast cancer. Although commonly used war metaphors crop up in her prose, the dominant and revolutionary theme is that any silence is a form of violence. As she explains, "I think of what this means to other Black women living with cancer, to all women in general. Most of all I think of how important it is for us to share with each other the powers buried within the breaking silence about our bodies and our health, even though we have been schooled to be secret and stoical about pain and disease. But that stoicism and silence does not serve us nor our communities, only the forces of things as they are" (*Burst* 118–119). To countenance the status quo in any arena in the Reagan-Bush era—or any era for that matter—certainly would have been uncharacteristic for Lorde. The layering of the silences she sought to extract from her body and other women's bodies was as complex and dense as the layers of tissues beneath her flesh. The way in which people are taught to be silent about the pain in their bodies is not altogether different from the way in which people learn to ignore segregation and racist violence.

Grounding the history of black women's inability to control their own bodies in the present-day context of cancer and apartheid made

Lorde's writing transformative, in part through the diary entries contained within *A Burst of Light*. Although breast cancer recurrence often translates into one's taking an inward, reflective stance on one's own mortality, Lorde reframed personal questions of survival and death as questions about the urgent crisis of apartheid. In this way she allowed readers into her quotidian existence so they could see just as much of what goes into the process of organizing for social change as of what goes into challenging the dominant Western cancer treatments.

For instance, one of the essays grouped in *A Burst of Light* teaches black women activists how to organize across differences of sexuality, and in some ways her diary entries in the essay provide a model of how one works with and through differences in race, sexuality, language, class, nationality. Organizing women of the African diaspora—especially to dismantle the Afrikaner regime—proved to be a source of strength and courage for Lorde in multiple ways. In the summer of 1986 she traveled with the Zamani Soweto Sisters from South Africa to Bonnieux in southern France. She explained how antiapartheid organizing taught her how to appropriate various coping mechanisms to fight her cancer: "I learn tremendous courage from these women, from their laughter and their tears, from their grace under constant adversity, from their joy in living which is one of their most potent weapons, from the deft power of their large, overworked bodies and their dancing, swollen feet" (*Burst* 101).

While in France Lorde gave birth to one of the most fascinating aspects of *A Burst of Light*: she gracefully bears witness for South African women living under a repressive regime, broadening their stories for a wider U.S.-based feminist audience. She begins this process by setting the stage with a poetic description of their surroundings:

> I am sitting in the stone-ringed yard of Les Quelles, a beautiful old reclaimed silk factory, now a villa. Gloria and the women of the Zamani Soweto Sisters surround me, all of us brilliant and subtle under the spreading flowers of a lime-tea tree. It looks and feels like what I've always imagined the women's compound in some African village to have been, once. Some of us drink tea, some are sewing, sweeping the dirt ground of the yard, hanging clothes in the sunlight at the edge of the enclosure, washing, combing each other's hair. Acacia blossoms perfume the noon air as Vivian tells the stories behind the tears in her glowing amber eyes. (*Burst* 101)

As Vivian's interlocutor, Lorde takes in the harrowing narratives and with her words and images she sews a tapestry of pain that seems incongruous against the backdrop of the lovely summer day.

In Lorde's retelling, Vivian's stories are a twice-removed *testimonio* of the suffering and torture experienced under South African apartheid. In fact the bulk of this particular diary entry, dated June 21, 1986, reads like a *testimonio* on behalf of those who are silenced, who cannot publicly speak and narrate their experiences themselves. Indeed, by the very act of Lorde's committing these stories to memory by placing them in her published journal she intervenes in and connects the distorted history and the present of South Africa. In this sense, George Yúdice's definition of the *testimonio* aptly applies to her work: "an authentic narrative, told by a witness who is moved to narrate by the urgency of a situation (e.g., war, oppression, revolution, etc.). Emphasizing popular, oral discourse, the witness portrays his or her own experience as an agent (rather than a representative) of a collective memory and identity. Truth is summoned in the cause of denouncing a present situation of exploitation and oppression or in exorcising and setting aright official history" (44).[9] And this was precisely Lorde's objective on behalf of these women within the context of bearing witness to her own struggles with her illness.

As the diary entry—one of the longest in the book—progresses, the stories become more detailed and the victims begin to have names and more fully fleshed out contexts. The narratives of Ruth, Thembi, Petal, Emily, Linda, Mariah, Sofia, Etta, Rita, Helen, Bembe, Hannah, Mary, and Wassa are not stories of isolated incidents. Their experiences transform Lorde—and the reader—to such an extent that in the midst of listening to their stories she becomes struck by their presence: "Gentle, strong, beautiful—the women of Soweto imprint their faces and their courage upon me" (*Burst* 102). In each of their stories a woman's body takes center stage. Each one features a woman—and sometimes her children—whose body is tortured or who experienced violence at the hands of a state.

Most of the women's narratives are mediated through Lorde's voice; however, she quotes three women directly. One of these women, Sula, calls attention to the more subtle forms of violence at the hands of Western Christian missionaries whose deceitful practices likely led to dangerous and unhealthy lifestyle choices. Through Lorde, Sula exposes the hypocrisy inherent in some of the contradictory and misleading messages the missionaries gave them: "'The missionaries lied to us so much about our bodies,' she said, indignantly, 'telling us they were dirty and we had to cover them up, and look now who is running about in bikinis on the Riviera, or naked and topless!'" (*Burst* 103). Although she does not say specifically what she was told about her body, and Lorde does not speculate, the underlying message is clearly racist: black bodies are inherently dirty and thus necessarily susceptible to disease, while white bodies are clean and healthy even as white people tan their flesh to make it appear temporarily darker. Implicit too in Sula's direct testimony is the need to cover up one's body—in other words, to silence it. Shrouding one's body in this sense resonates with the messages nurses and the ACS volunteers gave Lorde when they forced her to wear a lamb's wool puff in her bra.

Collecting these *testimonios* and presenting them in published form was one of the ways in which Lorde committed herself to end silences by speaking corporeal truths. The power of language loomed even larger when she explained that the Zamani Soweto Sisters engaged in subversive activities like placing "a tiny ANC [African National Congress, the anti-apartheid party] flag stitched on the little dead boy's pocket in the corner of a funeral procession quilt" (*Burst* 104). Quilting became yet another way for women to collectively resist silence as a conscious survival strategy. And Lorde engaged in this process because writing down these narratives and circulating them was akin to stitching together the funeral-procession quilt. Moreover, these stories did not end when they were laid down in print. Rather, this was merely the first step in transforming silence into language and action. Thus, at the end of the diary entry Lorde remarks: "There is work to be done" (*Burst* 106). That brief, simple sentence feels unbearably heavy for one woman. But Lorde did not intend for her words to lie listlessly on the page. This is her call. She expects her readers to join in and participate whenever there are silences to undo.

Telling stories of women suffering in Soweto is one way that Lorde saw herself as being of use. Another way was by telling her story about living with metastatic cancer. These two entities, as I have been arguing, were woven together. Lorde's writing about cancer cannot be extracted from the antiracist work she performs. She explains:

> Women who have asked me to set these stories down are asking me for my air to breathe, to use in their future, are courting me back to

my life as a warrior. Some offer me their bodies, some their enduring patience, some a separate fire, and still others, only a naked need
whose face is all too familiar. It is the need to give voice to the complexities of living with cancer, outside the tissue-thin assurance that
they "got it all," or that the changes we have wrought in our lives
will insure that the cancer never reoccurs. And there is a need to give
voice to living with cancer outside of that numbing acceptance of
death as a resignation waiting after fury and before despair. There is
nothing I cannot use somehow in my living and my work, even if I
would never have chosen it on my own, even if I am livid with fury
at having to choose. (*Burst* 111)

The way in which embodied images arise from this passage is important
because they guide our thinking about cancer and racism. Lorde supports this metaphoric contention further down in the passage: "Racism.
Cancer. In both cases, to win the aggressor must conquer, but the resisters need only survive. How do I define that survival and on whose
terms?" (*Burst* 111). Embedding her own stories within narratives of
women whom she encountered in her political life and work makes
them inseparable. This gesture suggests a dialogic relationship across these
embattled experiences so that various groups of women may seek out
multiple methods of survival.

Sula's story certainly resonates with Lorde's trying to have agency in
the medical system. Making choices about what happens to her body
"not because I know more than anybody else, but simply because it is my
body" is a fundamental concern of Lorde's (*Burst* 118).[10] Metabolized
into the tissues of her body were the stories of many black women who
had not been able to make any choices about their bodies in a medical
arena or in any other arena. So when she contemplated choices about
her health, she considered the situations of historically enslaved black
women of the Americas and of the then–currently oppressed women under apartheid who could not make any bodily decisions.

Lorde's reiteration of political and bodily analogies seems designed
to ensure that her ideas puncture the skin of readers so that they will be
moved by an empathic response to this pain. She modeled this method of
being in the world when she showed readers how she made choices
about how to treat her body in the medical sphere and how she made

choices about how to react to violence against people of color. She made this link explicit: "So when I do a . . . reading to raise funds for the women's collectives in Soweto, or to raise money for Kitchen Table: Women of Color Press, I am choosing to use myself for things in which I passionately believe. When I speak to rally support in the urgent war against apartheid in South Africa and the racial slaughter that is even now spreading across the U.S., when I demand justice in the police shot-gun killing of a Black grandmother and lynchings in Northern Califor-nia and in Central Park in New York City, I am making a choice of how I wish to use my power" (*Burst* 119). That Lorde thought about power and choice in these contexts so cogently and that she so closely linked them together make it evident that her language indeed led to empow-ering decisions that were sometimes about herself but more often than not could heal others she worked to support and give voice to.

The above catalogue of globally situated, racist events that Lorde re-sisted while encouraging others to join her strikes a visceral chord, in part, because it fits into a historical and current pattern of physically and verbally silencing and wounding bodies of the African diaspora. Whether visible or not, violent injustices are palpable. Hortense Spillers explains that this history of enslaving and wounding black bodies leaves "undeci-pherable markings on the captive body [which] render a kind of hiero-glyphics of the flesh whose severe disjunctures come to be hidden to the cultural seeing by skin color. We might well ask if this phenomenon of marking and branding actually 'transfers' from one generation to an-other, finding its various *symbolic substitutions* in an efficacy of meanings that repeat the initiating movements?" (67). Concurring with Spillers, I would argue that these markings are transferred from one generation to the next. They can be transmitted through narrative, cautionary tales, and the like, which are then internalized beneath the layers of skin. Thus, when Lorde sought out the company of other brown-skinned women with whom she could commiserate and commune, she in part desired others who felt both the scar of their upper torso and all that scars on black bodies suggest historically.

It should come as no surprise, then, that when faced with being cut open a second time, Lorde responded with terror. Indeed, at several points in her narrative Lorde used the word *terror* to describe her fear of the standard medical modalities in the United States. But whenever she used this language, she conjured up the narratives of racist histories and apartheid, which permeate her skin, mind, and text. Many of these markings are undecipherable as Spillers suggests, but others are as tangible and visible as an encoded hieroglyphics that only Lorde can translate. Cutting open her skin felt like a violent action to her—whatever the context—in part because of the historical weight that scars carried for her. Whether her fear stemmed from her own mastectomy or from her ancestral past, the stories she listened to about apartheid played a role here. If, as Alexander suggests, "witnessing can be aural as well as ocular," then scars Lorde saw and stories she heard contributed to her decision to avoid being cut open in the face of metastasis ("Can" 85) because being cut and scarred registered as a part of the history of the torture and abuse of black people's bodies. As Lorde described her reaction to a second round of surgery, racism and cancer figured as almost interchangeable metaphors: "If this is cancer and they cut me open to find out, what is stopping that intrusive action from spreading the cancer or turning a questionable mass into an active malignancy?" (*Burst* 113–114). This specific questioning of cancer treatment relied on language—intrusive—that resonated with the way history marked her corporeally. The terror came from feeling as though she had no power or control over her body in this medical setting.

These feelings occasioned Lorde's sense that in order to translate her bodily fear into language and action she should publish this diary. And that decision interrupted the writing process even as new cancer growth interrupted her life. Therefore, in a metatextual insertion, she tells readers that she needs to lay out how she learned about her metastasis and how she chose to treat it; and, accordingly, midway through her diary-essay, on November 8, 1986, Lorde backtracks. Her diary entries begin to narrate the story of her cancer in retrospect rather than observing the moment or experiences from the day recorded at the top of the page. All this recursive narration facilitates her move to regain control over her life, body, and story.

Healing began, for Lorde, when she took control of her body by imagining connections between what went on inside her body and what went on outside her body. Linking two wars—one against global forms of racism and the other against cancer cells spreading through her body—led her to question the status quo and normative institutional powers and practices. In the epilogue to *A Burst of Light* she reflects on how she tackled healing in this respect:

> I visualize daily winning the battles going on inside my body, and this is an important part of fighting for my life. In those visualizations, the cancer at times takes on the face and shape of my most implacable enemies, those I fight and resist most fiercely. Sometimes the wanton cells in my liver become Bull Conner and his police dogs completely smothered, rendered impotent in Birmingham, Alabama by a mighty avalanche of young, determined Black marchers moving across him toward their future. P. W. Botha's bloated face of apartheid squashed into the earth beneath an onslaught of the slow rhythmic advance of furious Blackness. Black South African women moving through my blood destroying passbooks. (*Burst* 132–133)

These images are quite powerful and forceful. She used these political battles as weapons to fight her cancer because, as she says, "Cancer itself has an anonymous face. When we are visibly dying of cancer, it is sometimes easier to turn away from the particular experience into the sadness of loss, and when we are surviving, it is sometimes easier to deny that experience. But those of us who live our battles in the flesh must know ourselves as our strongest weapon in the most gallant struggle of our lives" (*Burst* 133). It is as if the exchange of *testimonio* with the South African women sealed a nurturing, sustaining bond that moved metaphorically inside Lorde's flesh and traveled through her body. Communal, narrative energy fueled Lorde's agency in surviving cancer just as her collection of *testimonios* enabled the women's survival under apartheid.

LANGUAGE

With her strong political and emotional commitments to fighting for her life and for her kin living under apartheid—at home in the Americas and abroad in South Africa—Lorde organized a conference in St. Croix with Sojourner Sisters; at the conference she experienced "the real power of a small group of women of the Diaspora in action" (*Burst* 97). In St. Croix much of her work about herself and others merged: the anniversary of a friend's mastectomy, the death of South African writer Ellen Kuzwayo's sister from breast cancer, and ultimately the birth of Sisterhood in Support of Sisters in South Africa (SISA). Through these experiences Lorde found new ways to unpack and rethink the political forces working against people living under apartheid as well as people living with cancer. Although race certainly colored this view for Lorde, she also knew that the economic component was a crucial part of the puzzle. She asks, "What would it be like to be living in a place where the pursuit of definition within this crucial part of our lives was not circumscribed and fractionalized by the economics of disease in america? Here the first consideration concerning cancer is not what does this mean in my living, but how much is this going to cost?" (*Burst* 99).

Thinking about the systemic role of cancer in her body led her to consider broader connections between cancer and the environment; the way cancer functions parallels the systemic ways in which racism functions in the world. In this context, in light of these struggles, Lorde explained what it meant and why it was imperative to put her body on the line on behalf of herself and those whose lives she fought for: "It takes all of my selves working together to effectively focus attention and action against the holocaust progressing in South Africa and the South Bronx and Black schools across this nation, not to speak of the streets. Laying myself on the line. It takes all of my selves working together to fight this death inside me. Every one of these battles generates energies useful in the others" (*Burst* 99). Rather than approach cancer with dread Lorde channeled her fear into something useful. When she spoke of being of use in the world, she enacted this practice inside and outside her body. The streets in which she placed her body on the line were analogous to the avenues in her body through which this political nerve traveled. Thus, the dialogic energy that moved between her political and medical battles informed each contest. Moreover, her political questioning provided her with tools to dissect this medical maze. And this set of burgeoning analyses between corporate and state powers, the medical establishment, racism, sexism, homophobia, and the environment proved to be the most revolutionary aspect of the agency she acquired to heal herself. The legacy of that healing, in turn, was passed onto generations of women with breast cancer who were influenced by her words.

Metastasis to the liver led Lorde to use death in a provocative way by urgently addressing global issues of mortality and pain affecting women of the African diaspora. This new phase of cancer also pushed Lorde to consider the relationship between her body and the earth; and these musings compelled her to consider innovative healing modalities. In each instance, Lorde maintained agency in the process, building on the legacy of Kushner as well as heeding the call of Carson. In the United States her doctors transparently tried to control her body and make decisions for her despite the fact that the radiological tests they ran were inconclusive. In a characteristic response to them, and much to their dismay, she said, "They refuse to look for any other reason for the irregularities in the x-rays, and they're treating my resistance to their diagnosis as a personal affront. But it's my body and my life and the goddess knows I am paying enough for all this, I ought to have a say" (*Burst* 76). Lorde reiterated her desire and demand for a choice and a voice when it came to making decisions about her body whether that meant she did not wear a prosthesis or did not have a liver biopsy.

Thinking uniquely about the world and her body turned Lorde to alternative medicine. While in Berlin she began treatment with an anthroposophic doctor, in part because "they believe in surgery only as a last resort" (*Burst* 58). But given Lorde's approach to her body and mind it is likely that she committed herself to this modality, developed by Rudolf Steiner, because it relied heavily on using the mind to heal the body cognitively and spiritually.[11] Iscador injections—"a biological made from mistletoe which strengthens the natural immune system and works against the growth of malignant cells"—became one of the holistic medicinal approaches to cancer that she relied on (*Burst* 59).[12] In November 1985, Lorde learned that the mass on her liver was spreading despite the appearance of improvement as a result of the Iscador. In order to continue her anthroposophic medical treatments, Lorde traveled with Frances to the Lukas Klinik in Switzerland to participate in a research trial of Iscador and to receive treatment in a holistic medical setting.

The change of venue forced Lorde to consider what it meant for her to treat her body and mind holistically and to think about the planet in a similar vein. Being present in her body in a particularly reflective way on New Year's Day in 1986, Lorde suggested profound links between the various struggles for survival that women of the African diaspora face:

Today Frances and I hiked to the top of a mountain to see the Dornach ruins, and the whole Rhine valley spread out beneath us. It felt so good to be moving my body again. My mother always used to say that whatever you do on New Year's Day you will do all year round, and I'd certainly like to believe that's true. It was very cold and sunny and bright, three miles up and back. The ruins rang with that historical echo and the presence of trials labored and past, although not as profoundly as the stones of El Morro in Cuba, and certainly not as desperately as the walls of Elmina Castle in Ghana, from whence so many Black women and children and men were sent to hell—slavery. (*Burst* 94)

At the same time, the striking beauty of the land with a backdrop of an infernal trauma reflected Lorde's body: although she embraced her scar and viewed her postmastectomy body with affection, the scar resurrected memories of wounding, of cutting. This fear of being cut open again—a fear of the knife itself as well as a fear of the knife's ability to agitate the cancer cells and assist in their proliferation through her internal organs—motivated Lorde to seek treatment at the Lukas Klinik. At the time, in the United States questioning chemotherapy was as radical as refusing to wear a prosthesis. In Europe, this was not exactly the case. In any event, asking difficult and previously unasked questions was par for the course for Lorde.

Too, weaving together what might have seemed like otherwise disparate subjects also came almost naturally to her. For instance, she suggested links between covering up the surface of a one-breasted body and covering up the use of carcinogenic materials that corporations manufacture and sell to the public. In one of her most powerful polemic moments, she argued, "My scars are an honorable reminder that I may be a casualty in the cosmic war against radiation, animal fat, air pollution, McDonald's hamburgers and Red Dye No. 2, but the fight is still going on, and I am still a part of it. I refuse to have my scars hidden or trivialized behind lambswool or silicone gel" (*Cancer* 61). Even in *The Cancer Journals,* Lorde begins to link silencing the body to repressing subjects in dominant discourse within various public spheres. Like Carson before her, Lorde wonders about the politics behind these taboo subjects.

Indeed, in *The Cancer Journals* the narrative increasingly points to the environment as a cause of cancer and as the arena in which prevention research must occur. As Lorde moves through the text that perspective becomes more strongly asserted. And, clearly, she amplifies that argument in *A Burst of Light*. For the last month of diary entries, recorded in November and December 1986, Lorde puts forward her argument about the role oppression plays in environmentally caused cancer. "I do not find it useful any longer to speculate upon cancer as a political weapon. But I'm not being paranoid when I say my cancer is as political as if some CIA agent brushed past me in the A train on March 15, 1965 and air-injected me with a long-fused cancer virus. Or even if it is only that I stood in their wind to do my work and the billows flayed me. What possible choices do most of us have in the air we breathe and the water we must drink?" (*Burst* 120).[13]

These questions present a perspective that was sorely lacking in the late 1980s. The way in which Lorde politicized breast cancer takes bodies and the environment into account. Cancer is political not because either subject—bodies or the environment—is inherently political, but rather because of the silence and secrecy surrounding the overlapping intersections of these subjects. About this type of political repression, Eisenstein makes it clear that issues are necessarily racially and economically inflected: "Environmental devastation and hazards are most often silenced and with them their racial and class aspects are smothered as well. Pesticides and industrial pollutants are treated as inevitable, and naturalized as part of our landscape as such. There is a faint recognition that poorer people, living in areas closer to industry and its pollution, suffer these consequences more directly" (72). Eisenstein indicates the cycle of pollution and cancer by highlighting our own complicity and silence about the way environmentally linked cancer gets naturalized.

One way that Lorde attempted to interrupt that cycle was to use what seemed like natural products to treat her illness without dissociating the mind from the body. Although the regimen for the patients at the Lukas Klinik appeared to be open and healing, she discovered that even this spiritually motivated medicine—particularly this brand of rigidly Christian-focused healing—could be "dogmatic" (Lorde, *Burst,* 82). Instead of submitting her body to a surgeon, she practiced "Curative Eurhythmy with a tiny East Indian woman named Dilnawaz who was raised in Rudolf Steiner schools in India.... [Curative Eurhythmy] is a combination of sustained rhythmical body movements and controlled breathing, based upon vowel and consonant sounds" (*Burst* 82). This aspect of healing, because of its reliance on the body, mind, and language, which Dilnawaz emphasized, seemed in line with her body's natural healing potential, a philosophy that is a fundamental component of anthroposophy. Dilnawaz, the only woman of color in a sea of white faces, reminded Lorde of this most vital aspect of this type of healing: "The treatment of any disease, and of cancer in particular, must be all of a piece, body and mind, and I am ready to try anything so long as they don't come at me with a knife" (*Burst* 83). Listening to her body and believing in these homeopathic remedies enabled Lorde to cultivate tools for fighting cancer in ways that gave her agency. Making certain she researched this situation and thought it through intellectually while paying attention to her body's needs gave her a role in this process. But it was a process of constant questioning. She revealed her uncertainty and hesitation after she received a definitive diagnosis of liver cancer: "Iscador or chemotherapy or both?" (*Burst* 89).

Although she does not mention specifically what she believes caused her cancer in *A Burst of Light* or *The Cancer Journals*, her labor in one particular factory as a young woman foreshadowed a later cancer diagnosis. She describes this episode in *Zami: A New Spelling of My Name*, her biomythography, which she wrote between her autobiographical prose texts specifically about cancer.[14] In this fictionalized autobiography, she tells about her exposure to carcinogenic materials while working for Keystone Electronics in Stamford, Connecticut. The factory, which she describes as "Dante's Inferno," employed mostly blacks and Puerto Ricans from New York City. The labor involved, among other activities, "reading crystals on a variety of X-ray machines, or wash[ing] the thousands and thousands of crystals processed daily in huge vats of carbon tetrachloride" (*Zami* 126). Had Lorde written this book without the specter of cancer—and her publicness about it—perhaps the chapters about a young Lorde working in factories would have read quite differently. But in addition to describing the people working at the factory and the labor they performed, she also inserts a postcancer perspective when she theorizes about the environmental hazards that workers of color were subjected to: "Nobody mentioned that carbon tet destroys the liver and causes cancer of the kidneys. Nobody mentioned that the X-ray machines, when used unshielded, delivered doses of constant low radiation far in excess of what was considered safe even in those days. Keystone

Electronics hired Black women and didn't fire them after three weeks. We even got to join the union" (*Zami* 126).

This factory scene and the environmental racism implicit in it, in a sense, signals a moment in her diary in which Lorde encounters a fellow patient, a white, elderly schoolteacher who had also worked in a toxic environment as a young woman. In both cases working-class women were forced into factory work, where they were exposed to toxic materials. The significant difference is that the elderly schoolteacher's xenophobia led her to expose herself to carcinogenic matter whereas Lorde was subjected to lethal material without being warned by the corporation. In this episode, Lorde synthesizes some connections among racism, cancer, and the environment when this woman intrudes on an intimate tea she and Frances are having on a day off in the village of Arlesheim. The woman clings to Frances and Audre because she is alone and has found out that her breast cancer has metastasized to her bones (*Burst* 92). The story of how she likely acquired her breast cancer is most compelling because of all it says at the crossroads of race, class, and environmental contaminants. Lorde retells her story:

> She and her sister had had to live with foreign workers (she meant Italians) in the factory where they worked during World War II, and . . . the foreigners were very dirty, with lice and fleas, so she and her sister would sprinkle DDT in their hair and their beds every night so as not to catch diseases! And she is sure that is why the cancer has spread to her bones now. There was something so grotesque about this sad lonely old woman dying of bone cancer still holding on to her ethnic prejudices, even when she was realizing that they were going to cost her her life. The image of her as a young healthy aryan bigot was at war inside me with the pathetic old woman at our table and I had to get out of there immediately. (*Burst* 92–93)

In *Zami* sometimes it seems as if the black and Puerto Rican workers are used as guinea pigs for cancer experimentation. And in fact this portion of Lorde's narrative, which occurs approximately halfway through the biomythography, becomes extremely tragic for those familiar with Lorde's body of work. Readers follow a young, poor Lorde desperate to acquire enough money to move to Mexico. This desperation leads her to cheat Keystone by appearing to speed up the crystal-count-ing process. She does this by slipping "crystals into my socks every time I went to the bathroom. Once inside the toilet stall, I chewed them up with my strong teeth and flushed the little shards of rock down the com-mode. I could take care of between fifty and a hundred crystals a day in that manner, taking a handful from each box I signed out" (*Zami* 146). Thus a desperate, if naive, Lorde has some agency in placing her body and its well-being on the line. In contradistinction, in *A Burst of Light* it is the elderly schoolteacher whose action necessarily, if ignorantly, causes her cancer (if we take Carson's arguments seriously).

ACTION

Deborah McDowell reminds us that "Lorde placed her body firmly on the line in everything she wrote, even and especially when it was be-ing ravaged by breast cancer" (310). Using her body as a way to testify to the silences surrounding black women's bodies in the healthcare arena provided a powerful model for writers and activists while providing a lesson for physicians and politicians. Her writing also left a deep imprint in several counterpublic spheres, and this impression has helped to widen the range of choices available to women with breast cancer, particularly women of color, lesbians, and poor women. Her work continues to speak to this last silence, which Carson, Ford, and Kushner left largely unbro-ken. Images of and allusions to Lorde saturate the literature of poets with cancer such as Pat Parker, Lucille Clifton, Alicia Ostriker, Eve Kosofsky Sedgwick, Marilyn Hacker, and June Jordan.[15] Her words inspire a variety of actions in several different contexts: her writing serves as a model for other women writing about their illness in narrative form and in self-help form; her ideas motivate people to consider new methods of treat-ment; her politics enable people to consider various modes of resistance to hegemonic ideas about women's bodies and women's health.

Even the most cursory glance through anthologies about breast can-cer, women's health, and women's bodies reveals that Lorde's *The Cancer Journals* and *A Burst of Light* continue to speak to women's concerns.[16] Other books, like Linda Villarosa's *Body and Soul*, Sharon Batt's *Patient No More,* and Midge Stocker's *Confronting Cancer, Constructing Change,* are dedicated to Lorde's memory. Primary feminist books about women's health, like Villarosa's, Deborah Hobler Kahane's *No Less a Woman,* and the Boston Women's Health Book Collective's *Our Bodies, Ourselves,* refer readers to Lorde's books in their bibliographies and as resources.

In other volumes of collected writing about cancer, many women refer specifically to Lorde's text as a way to pay homage to their own consciousness-raising process. Her work makes women feel safe to question standardized medical practices while encouraging them to continue her tradition of speaking out and ending silences about the disease. Sandra Steingraber, whose writing about breast cancer suggests that Lorde influenced her as much as Carson did, alludes to both women in poetry and prose. From Steingraber's poem "Apology to Audre Lorde, Never Sent" to her essays about environmental carcinogens, Lorde figures prominently in Steingraber's work as she reminds readers "to replace New Age heal-thyself concepts of disease prevention with political action" ("Lifestyles" 98). Elsewhere Steingraber claims that, "thus far, we have let Audre Lorde do too much of [the political work] by herself" ("We All" 45). She comes to this conclusion after reflecting on the diary entry in *A Burst of Light* in which Lorde comments on the chemical plants between Zurich and Basel. Steingraber argues that we must continue to challenge the unquestioned and sanctioned discourse about what causes cancer.

Still, it can be argued that only the literary and politically minded woman will find her way to the above-referenced texts. And although women stumbling on the title *The Cancer Journals* in the various bibliographies accompanying these works may be directed to Lorde's writing, it does not follow that her ideas will reach a broad base of women across categories of race, class, and sexuality. The one book that can help to make Lorde a household name for women with breast cancer, however, is *Dr. Susan Love's Breast Book.* In many respects a contemporary version of Kushner's *Breast Cancer,* this self-help manual was written by a white, lesbian, activist breast surgeon.[17] Love not only refers readers to Lorde's books, she also embeds quotations from Lorde's work within the body of her text. In keeping with themes important both to Kushner and to Lorde, Love uses the poet as an example of someone who chose not to have chemotherapy and instead chose Iscador as a way to encourage readers to make their own treatment decisions (293, 449). Love also quotes Lorde's famous sentiments about the ways in which prostheses keep women silent as a way to teach women about compulsory femininity (385).

Lorde's unflinching criticisms of and challenges to dominant modes of medical treatment for women continue to influence the medical community in other profound ways. Since her death on November 17, 1992, Lorde's legacy has survived outside of her literary work and within the medical arena in the form of the Michael Callen–Audre Lorde Community Health Center in New York City.[18] This center puts into operation Lorde's beliefs about healthcare by meeting the needs of gay men and lesbians. Next to her enlarged photograph in the lobby of the center is a quote from *The Cancer Journals:* "Every woman has a militant responsibility to involve herself actively with her own health. We owe ourselves the protection of all the information we can acquire. . . . And we owe ourselves this information *before* we may have a reason to use it" (75). Her memory is honored at this healthcare facility in two substantial ways. All members of the queer community, regardless of their ability to pay, can receive medical treatment; and the doctors help and encourage their patients to research standard and complementary treatment options in the center's Health Education Resource Center.

On the political stage Lorde's ideas have transformed and shaped the progressive arena, and they continue to do so with respect as much to feminist and antiracist politics as to the politics of health.[19] Certainly any account of Byllye Avery's National Black Women's Health Project in Atlanta would be remiss if it did not include Lorde's philosophy on the physical and emotional well-being of black women.[20] However, many of the links I suggest between Lorde's writing and politics and various political entities are implicit.[21] The exception is Breast Cancer Action (BCA) in San Francisco, which consistently makes explicit the myriad ways in which Lorde's legacy galvanizes its members. Barbara Brenner, the executive director of BCA, highlights Lorde's influence in many of the organization's monthly newsletters by quoting her work as a way to motivate women to act. In an article detailing the unique direct-action style of BCA, Brenner opens with an epigraph by Lorde and a reflection on her life: when Lorde was diagnosed there was no breast cancer movement; twelve years later, when she died, "breast cancer was no longer a personal secret; the breast cancer movement in the United States had grown from support groups to national organizations. Grass-roots groups were scattered across America" (325).

One of the ways in which BCA contributed to the burgeoning grass-roots breast cancer movement was to rename its direct-action task force the Audre Lorde Action Brigade. Formed in 1998 at a BCA town meeting, this group takes its inspiration from one particularly compelling activist statement that fuses the personal to the political:

> I would lie if I did not also speak of loss. Any amputation is a physical and psychic reality that must be integrated into a new sense of self. The absence of my breast is a recurrent sadness, but certainly not one that dominates my life. I miss it, sometimes piercingly. When other one-breasted women hide behind the mask of prosthesis or the dangerous fantasy of reconstruction, I find little support in the broader female environment for my rejection of what feels like a cosmetic sham. But I believe that socially sanctioned prosthesis is merely another way of keeping women with breast cancer silent and separate from each other. For instance, what would happen if an army of one-breasted women descended upon Congress and demanded that the use of carcinogenic, fat-stored hormones in beef-feed be outlawed? (*Cancer* 14–15)

What would happen indeed! BCA found out when it held its first Audre Lorde Action Brigade event to raise awareness about "the connection between pollution and cancer, cancer and corporate profits"; at this event women with mastectomies took off their shirts in the midst of San Francisco rush-hour traffic (Degen and Wilkinson).

Alluding to the power of such actions, Brenner explains why it is important to institutionalize Lorde's name whenever the BCA marches in public: "[My] reading—particularly of *The Cancer Journals* and *A Burst of Light*—inspired me to become a breast cancer activist. The passion of Audre Lorde's words and the clarity of her vision continue to inspire my activism and, in may ways, the work of BCA" ("From"). The BCA, one of the most politically radical breast cancer organizations in the United States, steadfastly questions and critiques the practices of the cancer establishment (the ACS, the NCI, pharmaceutical companies, medical researchers, and others who profit significantly from cancer patients) with the same force that Lorde did in her prose.

I conclude with these examples of how Lorde affects breast cancer literature, medicine, and politics to suggest that narrative text has an effect in the world. Like Carson, Ford, and Kushner before her, Lorde presented ideas that continue to resonate with women facing breast cancer who want answers to questions left unaddressed. And, as I suggested above, Lorde's work speaks not just to women with cancer. Her analyses of racism and apartheid, misogyny and homophobia, which she presents prophetically in her autobiographical work, can be extrapolated to other contexts both literary and political. And indeed her analyses generated new theories from Eisenstein, who traces links among race, class, gender, and the environment in ways that can extend Lorde's vision of ending silences. Using San Francisco as a case study, Eisenstein demonstrates the way these categories merge:

> african-american women in the Bay Area have the fourth-highest rate of breast cancer in the world. They, as well as most poor women, have to fight the . . . Social Services and Health Departments in order to get mammograms. They often are put on waiting lists for six to nine months. These same women have little access to experimental therapies and clinical trials or to major medical centers and research facilities. Although the trials themselves do not cost money, the follow-up care does. Women with out health insurance, or with insurance that does not pay for experimental procedures, have to have their own independent means. (96)

Eisenstein concludes that these factors, which for the most part often go unstudied, offer one explanation for the disparity between the incidence and mortality rates of white and black women.

In Jodi Flaws, Craig Newschaffer, and Trudy Bush's study of the discrepancies between black and white women's mortality and incidence rates, they discovered that between 1950 and 1992, the year Lorde died, white women's mortality remained "relatively stable while black women's mortality rates increased over time" (1008). This finding, they suggest, is of recent origin; they argue that one reason may be that "there have been differential changes in environmental exposures associated with breast cancer risk between black and white women" (1010). Most of the more recent literature reporting findings about race, socioeconomic status, and breast cancer unearth more questions than answers.[22]

With respect to socioeconomic status, it should be clear that this area needs to be further researched because the relationship between disease and health, in a global context, is always connected to class position. Nancy Krieger and Elizabeth Fee concur, arguing that "our patterns of health and disease have everything to do with how we live in the world. Nowhere is this more evident than in the strong social-class gradients apparent in almost every form of morbidity and mortality. Yet the lack of information and the conceptual confusion about the relationship between social class and women's health is a major obstacle. . . . In this country [the United States] we have no regular method of collecting data on socioeconomic position and health" (25).

Taking Lorde's writing as a cue should be useful to scientists who want to uncover the relationship of cancer, the environment, race, and class. Such studies would find, for instance, that some of the most toxic places in the United States are in the poorest neighborhoods, as Eisenstein points out. Scientists have begun to question the role of the environment in producing inequalities in breast cancer rates.[23] Women writing about breast cancer have put pressure on scientists and politicians to vocalize previously held silences. Whether Lorde contributed directly to the way science is evolving may not be detectable. However, those familiar with her words should find it impossible not to hear allusions to her polemical narratives in the transformation of breast cancer politics.

Conclusion

TAKING ACTION

READING AUDRE LORDE's breast cancer writing, which focuses as much on apartheid in South Africa as it does on her illness, one begins to wonder about women's health concerns in a global context. Racism and cancer intertwine, and each systemic disease provides her with a map with which to navigate the other. Economics, the environment, and medicine become layered into the way that she considers the systemic nature of each separately and combined. The breast cancer death of South African writer Ellen Kuzwayo's sister elicits much of her thinking about the economics of disease and the way in which breast cancer proliferates in a variety of toxic environments. Her placement of women's health issues in a global context complicates Rachel Carson's theories about the relationship between cancer and the environment by compelling us to consider the dynamics of race and socioeconomic status in that equation. Carson alerted us to the ways in which carcinogens travel in the air, water, and soil—and consequently in the food we eat and the air we breathe—and both women allude to the ways that we cannot control the paths those toxins take.

Given the various ways that carcinogens can travel through the atmosphere, it would seem that cancer would be a concern for women around the globe. In industrialized nations breast cancer incidence rates continue to rise. But in developing nations cancer is not even on the radar screen. Instead, diseases such as malaria, tuberculosis, and HIV/ AIDS plague countries in Asia and Africa where many women do not live to be old enough to develop breast cancer. In the December 2002 United Nations Population Fund report, women's health and environmental health were presented as two of the primary issues that the United Nations (UN), and indeed the world, must address.[1] These ideas were first articulated at the 1994 International Conference on Population and Development in Cairo, Egypt, which articulated a few key goals—"better reproductive health, universal education and gender equality, all within the context of human rights"—and their expected consequences—the eventual reduction of poverty and population in developing nations (Obaid 5). In the 2002 report, eight goals clearly indicate the priorities of the UN: eradicate extreme poverty and hunger; achieve universal primary education; promote gender equality and empower women; reduce child mortality; improve maternal health; combat HIV/AIDS, tuberculosis, malaria and other diseases; ensure environmental sustainability; develop a global partnership for development (Obaid 7). Paying attention to women's heath—including physical, intellectual, and emotional health—would mean reducing maternal and infant mortality rates. Creating sustainable environments would mean developing ways to protect it from contaminants.

The point from which each of the report's goals emerges is poverty. As the report explicitly states, "Poor health is a cause as well as an effect of income poverty" (Obaid 15). This vicious cycle has a tragic irony at its core: poverty and unsustainability in the global south arose out of Western colonialism, and the West is indifferent to epidemics that arise out of impoverished conditions in nations with predominantly brown-skinned people. Of the factors involved in the UN goals—population growth, mortality rates, women's health, and development—accessible, affordable reproductive healthcare and clean drinking water take precedence. Creating healthy, educated children ensures, to a certain extent, that they can become informed about issues like their health and their environment as they age. Survival in this report translates into something beyond what Lorde writes about in her journals. Here the concern is poverty with respect to the land as well as to its people. As Zillah Eisenstein cautions:

> As long as profit rather than health defines corporate priorities, we shall see more breast cancer across the globe because it is an effect of global capital's arrogance. As bodies are assaulted by the effects of war damage to the air and water, as chemical pollutants compromise people's immune systems, as dietary habits shift as part of global transformations in agriculture women will face new breast cancers. Breast cancer, more prevalent in postindustrial countries of the west

should be seen in part as a warning sign for the rest of the globe. And the late diagnosis of breast cancers in senegal, ghana, and other poor countries bespeaks another warning: that excessive poverty in African nations charts a different breast cancer scenario where mammograms, and radiation, and chemotherapies are beyond the reach of most women. (170)

And this is precisely Lorde's and Eisenstein's argument about the direction of research globally: cancer like all these diseases must be examined in conjunction with socioeconomic and environmental data.

Worldwide cancer incidence rates continue to rise, although they are highest in developed nations. According to a global epidemiological report, "The incidence is more modest in North Africa, South America, Eastern, Southeastern, and Western Asia, but it is still the most common cancer of women in these geographic regions" (Parkin et al. 49). To a certain extent, breast cancer mortality rates follow the incidence rates. However, the statistics reported do not take into account the fact that race and class determine the extent to which women have access to treatment, support, and screening. If these factors were included, they would compromise the U.S. claim to the highest global survival rates— 84 percent—in the NCI's Surveillance Epidemiology and End Results program. If more poor women and women of color were screened, incidence rates would go up, and survival rates would go down. Indeed, one of the most telling pieces of data in this study is the fact that breast cancer incidence rates increase when women migrate to the United States from countries like China and Japan, which enjoy some of the lowest rates in the world (Parkin et al. 50).[2] In other words, when women from China and Japan immigrate to the United States, their likelihood for acquiring breast cancer increases; moreover, with each succeeding generation, the chance for getting breast cancer increases as well.

Understanding the particularities of cancer incidence and mortality rates on a global scale is complicated because studies are published in multiple languages. But from non-U.S. medical articles written in English it is clear that research on breast cancer in other countries covers some of the same territory as it does in the United States. BRCA1 and BRCA2, the breast cancer genes, are being examined in China, Korea, India, and Saudi Arabia; the use of breast self-exam is being studied in

Iran and Jordan; and in Tanzania breast cancer doctors are comparing HIV/AIDS to breast cancer. This type of work is being done in addition to more generalized epidemiological work about breast cancer incidence and mortality rates. And, significantly, some studies focusing on environmental factors are being carried out in Colombia, where researchers are looking at the relationship between organochlorine exposure and breast cancer; and Palestinian and Israeli doctors are working on a collaborative project to determine the relationship between pesticide use and cancer. But it is difficult to gauge how much women in other countries discuss breast cancer among themselves. Are there support groups that meet in the privacy of women's homes or in community centers and hospitals?[3] Cultural and linguistic barriers also make it difficult to discern whether women are writing narratives about their experiences with breast cancer.

In the United States, however, women continue to write about breast cancer and the spaces where they choose to do so continues to expand. A brief Internet search on Google.com with the keywords "breast cancer" elicits a sea of information available to women who have the time, money, and resources to investigate their treatment and choose their own courses of action. Websites for national breast cancer organizations such as the National Alliance of Breast Cancer Organizations, Y-Me, the Susan G. Komen Breast Cancer Foundation, the National Breast Cancer Coalition, Breast Cancer Action (BCA), The Breast Cancer Fund, and the American Cancer Society are some of the first sites to come up. Although all these organizations perform political work, they also provide medical resources for patients who wish to know more about their illness.[4] And many of these sites have chat rooms or bulletin boards where women post their personal narratives and photographs. There are also a variety of medical-oriented resources on the Internet for women to explore; sites such as OncoLink.org (the Abramson Cancer Center at the University of Pennsylvania), Cancer.gov (the National Cancer Institute), and SusanLoveMD.com (created by the author of *Dr. Susan Love's Breast Book*) inform Internet surfers about clinical trials, treatment advances, support resources, and recent research; some sites even have chat rooms. For those women who prefer to treat their illness with more naturopathic remedies, Ann Fonfa, a breast cancer survivor/activist, started AnnieAppleseedProject.org, which is dedicated to sharing complementary therapies (prior to the Internet Fonfa distributed a pamphlet at breast cancer conferences).

For women without Internet access numerous books are available in bookstores and libraries, ranging from personal narratives to self-help manuals. Newsletters, like Harvard Medical School's *Women's Health Watch*, publish a great deal of material about the latest studies on breast cancer; most of the national breast cancer organizations also produce monthly newsletters; and there is also an entire magazine, *Mamm*, devoted to women with breast and ovarian cancer.

The widespread availability in the twenty-first century of a variety of publications and various methods for conducting research on one's illness amazes me. When my mother died in 1992 most of these resources were not available—at least not to the general public. Fortunately we lived close to UCLA, and she could go there to research the latest breast cancer treatments and options. But she generally had to comb through journal articles, which are often written in medical jargon. Sifting through this material she found herself drawn to an experimental stem-cell bone-marrow transplant with high-dose chemotherapy. Although her doctors guided her through this decision, she still needed to devote time to researching cutting-edge treatment. But because she didn't have the appropriate training in statistics and biology, it was challenging for her to become an informed consumer. The new forums realize they have a different audience than medical journals do. Addressing consumers— and indeed the shift in terminology from *patient* to *consumer* is remarkable—in magazines, websites, books, newsletters means using lay language to communicate treatment options. Often women's experiences are incorporated into the text as a way to validate medical claims. I know that my mother would have used these materials to determine which would be the best course of action for her. I often wonder in what ways these new tools would have made a difference in her life.

All these changes in information technology and greater access to and openness about breast cancer treatment do not necessarily translate into helpful advice. More material is available, physicians are more open—increasingly many of them are women and women of color—and yet in some ways women are still left in the dark. For instance, major studies relating to breast cancer—about the dangers of hormone replacement

therapy (HRT), about genetic links to breast cancer, and about the incidence rate of breast cancer on Long Island—have left many women confused. The studies published in prominent journals such as the *New
England Journal of Medicine* often get picked up by newspapers and are
eventually disseminated through sound bites on the evening news. This
ever-narrowing process often simplifies the complexity of the findings.
Thanks to women like Rose Kushner, Audre Lorde, and Betty Ford
women may have more options, but the decisions are much more difficult
to make.

One of the areas where breast cancer risk gets miscommunicated
falls under the umbrella of family history and heredity. Since the mapping of the first breast cancer gene (BRCA1 and later BRCA2), discovered by Mary-Claire King in 1990 and later cloned by Mark Skolnick,
the general public has come to see breast cancer as a genetic disease,
although less than 10 percent of women with breast cancers have inherited it.[5] Moreover, because many of the initial studies on BRCA1 and
BRCA2 recruited subjects in synagogues, researchers drew conclusions
about Jewish women of Ashkenazi descent that indicated they had higher
rates of breast cancer than other women. The problems with this research
became clear when questions about genetic testing emerged. Critics of
testing programs, like Susan Love, questioned what happens to women
whose insurance companies deny them coverage because they determine
breast cancer to be a preexisting condition. If a woman finds out that she
has the gene, even though that does not necessarily mean she will later
develop breast cancer, should she have a bilateral prophylactic mastectomy? An oophorectomy (removal of the ovaries)? In addition, members
of the Jewish community scrutinized these proposals and issues most
clearly because for some taking a genetic test and becoming a medical
guinea pig resonated too closely with medical experimentation in Nazi
Germany. The conclusions also contained some flaws, as Barron Lerner
points out: "Despite these mutations, Ashkenazi Jewish women did not
have higher rates of breast cancer than other groups of women" (*Breast
Cancer* 282).

To read the headlines in newspapers like the *Wall Street Journal* about
prophylactic mastectomy, one might conclude that if a woman has a family history of breast cancer, removing her breasts will reduce her risk by
90 percent. Indeed, in one case, although the *Journal* reported accurately

on a study by Lynn Hartmann and colleagues that was published in 1999 in the *New England Journal of Medicine,* the newspaper wrote about the results of the study as a positive finding without examining any of the negative aspects of this surgical measure (Langreth). In addition, according to Lerner, who analyzed the results of the study, "Eighteen lives had theoretically been saved by the mastectomies, [but] 619 other women who had agreed to removal of both breasts would have survived without the surgery. Therefore, prophylactic breast removal had actually saved the lives of less than 3 percent of women who had chosen this dramatic intervention" (*Breast Cancer* 287). In other words, Lerner suggests that most of the women who survived would have done so whether they had chosen to have the surgery or not. Moreover, as Jane Zones illustrates, one must pay attention to the economic implications of any medical procedure or finding: "Statistics are also used to exaggerate benefits. Rates of prophylactic mastectomy are surging because [of] the widespread and successful marketing of BRCA genetic susceptibility testing. The drastic option of amputating healthy breasts has been held out as an option for women at high risk of developing breast cancer" (128). Zones's critique is reminiscent of Kushner's and Lorde's writing and is an indication of how they might respond if they were still alive.

Eisenstein, who had breast cancer and who comes from a family with an extensive history of breast cancer encourages us to view the illness through a complex lens, as being "more socially, economically, and racially constructed than . . . genetically inherited. This means understanding a range of social factors: an increased number of women being exposed to toxicity in the workplace, shifting discourses about women's health, so-called science narratives with their masculinist and racialized assumptions, and global capital with its petro/chemical-pharmaceutical empire and postindustrial-medical complex" (85–86). In other words, having a genetic or familial connection to breast cancer does not mean that one will necessarily develop the disease. But the Western model for scientific research does not allow enough space for examining the various economic, environmental, and social aspects of disease.

Some of the same concerns that genetic testing and prophylactic mastectomy raise can be seen in the results of the Women's Health Initiative (WHI) study about HRT. In the summer of 2002, researchers halted this randomized controlled trial because the health risks outweighed the hypothesized benefits; in particular they found that taking estrogen plus progestin increases breast cancer risk (Writing Group for the Women's Health Initiative Investigators). For years women active in counterpublic spheres published articles in newsletters warning of the danger of HRT. Given that a woman's relative risk of developing breast cancer is connected to her lifetime production of estrogen, it seems logical to be skeptical about the wonders of Premarin, an HRT brand, which is "the second most frequently prescribed medication in the United States and account[s] for more than $1 billion in sales, and 22.3 million prescriptions" (Fletcher and Colditz 366). But the information about risks does not get communicated to mainstream women nearly as easily as Premarin gets marketed to them. Suzanne Fletcher and Graham Colditz's carefully written editorial responding to the WHI study addresses not only their colleagues but also women who may read their report in the *Journal of the American Medical Association* in print or on-line. They pose practical questions such as "How should practicing clinicians and the millions of women taking an estrogen/progestin combination react to the unexpected and disquieting results of this study?" (367). After delineating the difference between absolute risk and relative risk, they answer that because women took HRT to begin with to prevent disease and because the study "provide[s] strong evidence that the opposite is happening for important aspects of women's health, even if the absolute risk is low[,] ... we recommend that clinicians stop prescribing this combination for long-term use" (367).[6]

Another area in which questions continue to plague researchers as well as women with breast cancer is environmental studies. Theories about the relationship between cancer and the environment date back to Carson's *Silent Spring*. In fact friends initially piqued her interest in the subject when they wrote to her about environmental contamination on Long Island, New York. Thirty years later, as women living in that region realized how many Long Island women were living with and dying from breast cancer, they formed an organization called 1 in 9 to raise awareness and study incidence rates. Using personal testimony, women pushed their representatives in Congress to initiate the Long Island Breast Cancer Study Project.[7] In 1993 the NCI and the National Institute of Environmental Health Sciences began their project in Nassau and Suffolk counties; in 2002 they released their initial results. The two case-control

studies of cancer incidence and environmental contaminants on Long Island examined the blood of women with and without breast cancer to
determine their exposure to organochlorine pesticides like DDT and
polychlorinated biphenyls (PCBs).[8] They found no links between breast
cancer and environmental toxins.

The results of this study swept through the mainstream news media
with a powerful force, and in most of these reports science writers accepted the results without question. One of the activists leading the challenge to this study was BCA's Barbara Brenner, who, in the spirit of
Carson and Lorde, pointed out its limitations. First, she argued that
rather than a case-control study "a study that follows subjects over a long
period of time—a longitudinal study—is much more likely to help us
understand the environmental factors contributing to breast cancer"
("Lessons" 2). Second, the project chose to look at pesticides and chemicals "that have long been banned from production and use in the United
States" ("Lessons" 2). Brenner suggests that following women with breast
cancer over the course of decades—as opposed to just seven years—and
focusing on environmental contaminants that are currently present on
Long Island would be a much better methodology to employ. And I
would add that such a longitudinal study should allow epidemiologists to
also collect data about race and socioeconomic status, which could provide significant insight into this disease.

When the *Journal of the National Cancer Institute* reported the news of
this study, it ran a sidebar column with a telling insight: "Activists were
kept out of the loop in deciding what kind of case-control study to do.
The lesson activists learned during this long study, they say, is that they
must stay on top of the research, and they also need to help direct it"
(Twombly 1349). Activists on Long Island had been voicing complaints
for a few years. Janette Sherman wrote about some of their quite serious
concerns about the inappropriate handling of blood samples a few years
prior to the publication of the study: "insufficient quantities drawn; clot-
ting of some samples; lack of coordination with environmental sampling;
and samples obtained from women after radiation and/or chemotherapy
treatment had begun" (181). Given these concerns, it would seem that a
model more closely related to the Silent Spring Institute's long-term
project, which blends the expertise of survivors and scientists, might
yield more accurate results while empowering the women whose health

depends on accurate research methods. And some of the geographical and environmental factors on Cape Cod apply to Long Island as well. Both places have a sole-source aquifer. As Sherman explains, "This means that all the water used by people living on Long Island lies, as in a pocket, under the land where they live, work, dump chemicals, apply pesticides, operate incinerators and nuclear facilities, and carry on the various activities of their lives. Rainfall carries the contaminants into an aquifer to mix and migrate throughout the water supply underlying the land" (52). Some of the materials released into the aquifer as well as the soil and air came from the Brookhaven National Laboratory "and the surrounding nuclear power plants" (Sherman 48).

Given the complexity of issues such as HRT, environmental links to breast cancer, as well as genetic testing and prophylactic mastectomy, it is easy to see how ordinary women might have a difficult time deciphering studies about breast cancer. There is much debate about each of these controversial issues, and there are no simple answers. On the one hand, greater openness about breast cancer doesn't equal better advice or access to treatment. On the other hand, increased openness has led to more research, which is now also focusing on groups of women who have historically higher mortality rates, such as African American women and Latinas. There is still much to be done, and few research projects have yielded any explicitly viable options. However, monitoring and educating women of color and poor women continues to be a project that women will benefit from in the long run—especially in areas that harbor toxic waste or environmental contaminants. More information, however, often produces conflicting reports, and women who do not have a background in science or medicine may have trouble deciphering the research that they now have access to. Nevertheless, the indispensable work of Carson, Ford, Kushner, and Lorde demonstrates how powerful women's voices can be when they use narrative to effect change. Indeed, if the women on Long Island continue to disseminate their stories to wider public audiences, they could ultimately ensure a larger role for patients in NCI-initiated studies.

Although this book tries to demonstrate the significant role of literature in raising consciousness in order to effect change in the United States, this movement should be thought of on a global scale. If we take Carson's and Lorde's words to heart, we must think about the global environmental consequences of toxic materials. In many ways their warnings now seem prophetic as Nuha al-Radi's account of Baghdad after the war in Iraq in the early 1990s reveals:

> Outlook Programme on the BBC says 300 tons of depleted uranium in the southern battle area in Iraq are causing horrendous defects, babies with no heads, no eyes—there are no computers to make an exact count. It has seeped through the earth into the water system, which means agriculture is also affected. What is on the ground can still be cleaned, but it's a very expensive exercise. What is in the air remains in the air blowing around. So it's a catastrophe for centuries to come. Hiroshima is still paying for its bombardment and we are far worse off. Both are victims of American technology. All the US soldiers who took part in the Gulf War, and who had shrapnel wounds, still show depleted uranium in their sperm. In the 250 "Gulf families," 60 percent of children have been born with congenital defects. So what of Iraq? (166–167)

This journal entry, dated January 14, 1996, echoes Carson's concerns in *The Sea around Us* and *Silent Spring*. Later writers like Lorde, Sandra Steingraber, Brenner, and Eisenstein continued the work of making people aware of the damaging long-term effects of carcinogenic material. With the continued use of carcinogenic materials that filter into the air, water, and soil we need to continue to address these concerns by writing, speaking, and acting in visionary ways about the future. This is the example that these writers and this history of writing about breast cancer in the United States leave us with.

NOTES

PREFACE

1. I later edited a selection of my mother's diaries and published them in an anthology where much of this quoted material comes from: Jane Gibbons-Knopf, "The War inside My Body."

2. Edelman's book had such an enormous impact that she received thousands of letters from other motherless daughters. She eventually published them in a collection: *Letters from Motherless Daughters.*

3. U.S. veterans who have been suffering from Gulf War Syndrome are also implicated in these findings. Although Gulf War Syndrome is not a synonym for cancer, both diagnoses are connected to the depleted uranium used during the war. See Linda McCauley et al., "Illness Experience of Gulf War Veterans Possibly Exposed to Chemical Warfare Agents."

INTRODUCTION: TELLING STORIES

1. For a historical look at the NBCC's evolution as well as its practices and policies, see Karen Stabiner's *To Dance with the Devil.* For an examination of the theory behind the NBCC's lobbying strategies, see Kay Dickersin and Lauren Schnaper's "Reinventing Medical Research."

2. For historical material on breast cancer surgery, see Daniel de Moulin's *A Short History of Breast Cancer* and James Olson's *Bathsheba's Breast.*

3. To be sure, some physicians treated prostate cancer with equal rigor, removing "the prostate gland, seminal vesicles, and a portion of the bladder. As with breast cancer, this operation was used even for tiny cancers incidentally discovered when an enlarged prostate was removed to relieve urinary obstruction. More often than not, men receiving a radical prostatectomy wound up incontinent of urine and impotent" (Lerner, *Breast Cancer,* 88). However, there were also physicians who viewed the breast as did one surgeon who claimed it was a "nonvital and functionless gland" (Lerner, *Breast Cancer,* 89).

4. For a brief historical perspective on this subject, see Sheryl Burt Ruzek and Julie Becker, "The Women's Health Movement in the United States."

5. Dreifus's book contains articles by two women who would become quite central to the breast cancer movement: Rose Kushner and Rita Arditti.

6. In the newest edition of *Our Bodies, Ourselves,* the Boston Women's Health Book Collective reflects on this problem, which is indicative of feminism more generally. The collective responds to the issue of racism within feminism by stating, "While it is exciting that this book stays alive, growing and changing, the process of becoming more inclusive has been painful and difficult at

times. Like many groups initially formed by white women, we have struggled against society's, and our own internalized, presumption that middle-class white women are representative of all women, and thus have the right to define women's health issues and set priorities. This assumption does a great injustice by ignoring and silencing the voices of women of color, depriving us all of hard-won wisdom and crucial, life-saving information. This time around, many more women of color have been involved in creating this edition, writing some of the chapters, editing, and critically reading every chapter in the book. During this process, tensions sometimes arose about what to include or leave out and how to frame certain issues. The resulting vigorous discussions have greatly enriched the book's content. But as in any organic process, some conflicts still remain to be resolved" (22). Among other changes, various editions now target specific populations. For instance, the book appears in over nineteen different languages. In the United States there are also different editions for lesbians, Latinas, and aging women. Eventually the women's health movement spawned texts that featured women of color. Books similar to *Our Bodies, Ourselves* and marketed to a mainstream audience focus specifically on the health needs of black women and Latinas. These texts encourage women of color to take control of their healthcare. See Linda Villarosa's *Body and Soul* and Jane Delgado's *¡Salud!,* which was simultaneously published in a Spanish-language edition.

7. Ann Landers, otherwise known as Dear Abby, also encouraged her audience to push for a war on cancer. She joined forces with the ACS and published letters and responses that demonstrated the powerful role government could have in the fight against cancer. "A Landers column to this effect in April 1971 unleashed such an avalanche of mail on Capitol Hill (Senator Alan Cranston of California said he received 60,000 letters) that congressional secretaries placed signs on their desks to 'Impeach Ann Landers'" (Patterson 248).

8. Let me be clear: I applaud the availability of alternatives to hormone-replacement therapy. My problem is with the appropriation of the term *feminist* in GlaxoSmithKline's marketing campaign, which I believe dilutes a term that should connote radical opposition to corporate consumer culture. Moreover, the relationship between pharmaceutical companies (like GlaxoSmithKline, the manufacturers of Remifemin), cosmetic corporations (like Avon and Estee Lauder), and breast cancer advocacy groups can potentially dilute the radical political impetus that was part of the breast cancer movement's origins (as evidenced in and maintained by groups like the Women's Community Cancer Project in Cambridge, Massachusetts, and Breast Cancer Action in San Francisco). Instead we have the opportunity for women to consume products like makeup or shoes to raise money for breast cancer research. Ellen Leopold calls attention to this contradictory situation: "The emphasis on consuming as a way of raising money— shopping for the cure—trades on the most conventional expectations of women rather than on their capacity for social action" ("Shopping" 6).

9. See Sandra Steingraber, "Lifestyles Don't Kill. Carcinogens in Air, Food, and Water Do."

CHAPTER 1   MISS CARSON GOES TO WASHINGTON

1. U.S. Congress, Senate Committee on Government Operations, 206.

2. Some of the texts that highlight Carson's effect on public policy and public health are Linda Lear's "Rachel Carson's *Silent Spring*," Frank Graham Jr.'s

Since Silent Spring, Helmut van Emden and David Peakall's *Beyond Silent Spring,* Gino Marco, Robert Hollingworth, and William Durham's *Silent Spring Revisited,* and James Whorton's *Before Silent Spring.*

3. U.S. Congress, Senate Committee on Government Operations, 220–221.

4. For her role as a government employee and her later struggles with the government to regulate pesticide use, see Linda Lear's "Bombshell in Beltsville."

5. Although her concern about pesticide spraying was not focused exclusively on its potential to increase cancer incidence, that perspective dominated her first public lecture on the subject for the Quaint Acres Community Association. She conducted most of her research on cellular biology and physiology at the National Cancer Institute (NCI) and the Library of Medicine. Her ideas were informed by the work of Wilhelm Heuper at the NCI. According to Robert Proctor, Heuper "was the most powerful American champion of the view that increased exposure to industrial chemicals was producing unprecedented levels of cancer" (36). Chemical corporations repeatedly tried to discredit Heuper's work; du Pont, for instance, "accused him of being a Nazi in the 1940s and a Communist in the 1950s—he was neither" (36).

6. Lear elaborates corporate criticisms of Carson: "First, Carson wrote for the public, a calling that somehow compromised her scientific credibility by implying that she was less than professional. She was an artist of acknowledged craft and merit, whose literary stock-in-trade was her ability to appeal to the public through their emotions. Point in fact: The opening fable [of *Silent Spring*] was almost uniformly derided by reviewers unable to understand its basis in allegory and [who] used it to demean her credibility as a scientist. Second, Carson was not a professional scientist. She had only a master's degree in zoology, had little field experience, held no academic appointment, and had not published in any peer-reviewed journals" (*Witness* 430).

7. Rachel Carson to Marjorie Spock and Polly Richards, 12 Apr. 1960, Rachel Carson Papers, Yale Collection of American Literature, Beinecke Rare Book and Manuscript Library, Yale University (hereafter RCP), quoted in Lear, *Witness,* 367.

8. To be sure, Carson was not the first to discover the toxic effects of DDT, nor was she the first to write about them. However, she was the first person to widely publicize and exhaustively document these concerns for a mass public audience. See Christopher Bosso's *Pesticides and Politics,* Thomas Dunlap's *DDT,* Clarence Cottam and Elmer Higgins's "DDT and Its Effect on Fish and Wildlife," Neil Hotchkiss and Richard Pough's "Effect on Forest Birds of DDT Used for Gypsy Moth Control in Pennsylvania."

9. For details about these legal threats, see Paul Brooks's *The House of Life.* Brooks was Carson's editor at Houghton Mifflin during the publication of *Silent Spring,* and much of his biographical work on her illustrates the various obstacles they faced while trying to get her message out to the public.

10. For an analysis of Carson from this perspective, see Sandra Steingraber's " 'If I Live to Be 90 Still Wanting to Say Something.' "

11. Both technologies were used abroad during the war and then used on civilians—without their knowledge—in the postwar era. For an extended analysis of these connections, see Ralph Lutts's "Chemical Fallout" and Pete Daniel's "A Rogue Bureaucracy."

12. This letter, "Mr. Day's Dismissal," *Washington Post,* 22 Apr. 1953, is reprinted in Carson, *Lost Woods,* 100. She protested the firing because it indicated to her the administration's suspicious policies on conservation.

13. Dorothy Freeman to Rachel Carson, 23 Jan. 1962, quoted in Freeman 395.
14. Rachel Carson to Dorothy Freeman, 1 Feb. 1958, quoted in Freeman 249.
15. Ibid., 248.
16. Dorothy Freeman to Rachel Carson, 23 Jan. 1962, quoted in Freeman 395.
17. For histories of romantic friendship and lesbianism, see Carroll Smith-Rosenberg's *Disorderly Conduct* and Lillian Faderman's *Surpassing the Love of Men*.
18. Rachel Carson to Dorothy Freeman, 6 Feb. 1954, quoted in Freeman 19–20.
19. Dorothy Freeman to Rachel Carson, 29 Feb. 1964, quoted in Freeman 529–530.
20. Lear explains that Carson's internist, Michael Healy, chose Sanderson and that Carson "was not much involved in discussions about the various outcomes. Perhaps Carson's casual attitude was the product of her absorption in her work, her past experience with benign cysts, or just an unwillingness to think about unpleasant possibilities. It was in keeping with her earlier response, but an attitude she later regretted" (*Witness* 558–559).
21. Michael Healy to George Crile Jr., 13 Dec. 1960, George Crile, Jr., Family Papers, Helga Sandburg Crile, Cleveland Clinic Foundation Archives [hereafter CFP], quoted in Lear, *Witness*, 367; emphasis mine. Carson later revealed, "If only I could set the calendar back two years. It was April 1 I entered the hospital. How differently I would handle it now—how carefully I would select the surgeon" (Rachel Carson to Dorothy Freeman, 28 Mar. 1962, quoted in Freeman 400).
22. Rachel Carson to Paul Brooks, 27 Dec. 1960, RCP, quoted in Lear, *Witness*, 368.
23. Rachel Carson to Dr. George Crile Jr., 7 Dec. 1960, CFP, quoted in Leopold, *A Darker*, 129.
24. Healy's letter to Crile stated: "Dr. Sanderson did not tell Miss Carson that she had a malignancy, but said that she had a condition bordering on a malignancy. Because of her being quite informed that there was no malignancy, her present management is quite difficult" (Michael Healy to George Crile, 13 Dec. 1960, CFP, quoted in Lear, *Witness*, 379).
25. Crile recommended that because Carson had not yet reached menopause she first "undergo sterilization by radiating the ovaries" (Lear, *Witness*, 379). By January 1961 Carson "was sterilized and started the first series of ten radiation treatments," which lasted through March (Lear, *Witness*, 380). Crile shared his recommendations with Healy in a letter offering his evaluation: "In the first place, I have discussed with her quite frankly what the situation is, pointing out that we view a tumor in lymph nodes as being a local disease and do not think that it should be treated at this stage with chemotherapy or with wide field radiation therapy" (George Crile to Michael Healy, 16 Dec. 1960, CFP, quoted in Lear, *Witness*, 379). He rationalized this decision by stating that, "at the time of Carson's illness, the NIH [National Institutes of Health] had just started its first clinical trial of a drug (thiotepa) designed specifically to control breast cancer, but Carson did not enroll in it. The absence of any of these drugs from Crile's armamentarium left him with hormone therapies as the only available treatments that could address Carson's cancer as a systemic disease rather than a local one" (Leopold, *A Darker* 131). James Patterson offers some insight into Crile's philosophy on radiation in a broader context: "Much radical surgery, they said, was not only unnecessary; it might even hasten metastasis. Studies in the late 1950s of breast cancer surgery suggested that

women who underwent simple removal of the breast followed by radiation
fared as well as women who endured radical mastectomies that also cut away
underlying muscles and auxiliary tissue. This counterattack stemmed the tide
of heroic surgery, but only slightly and slowly" (192). This rhetoric comes out
of the distinctions Crile made about the benefits of radiation as a therapeutic
treatment for breast cancer. Evidence suggested that radiation worked with
breast-conserving surgery as well as previous Halsted operations alone had.
Crile also operated in the post–World War II era, when radiology and oncology offered promise as therapies in addition to surgery.

26. Rachel Carson to Dorothy Freeman, 4 Jan. 1961, quoted in Freeman 327.
27. Rachel Carson to Dorothy Freeman, 17 Jan. 1961, quoted in Freeman 331.
28. Rachel Carson to George Crile Jr., 18 Mar. 1961, CFP, quoted in Leopold, *A Darker*, 136.
29. Rachel Carson to Dorothy Freeman, 17 Mar. 1961, quoted in Freeman 363.
30. Rachel Carson to Dorothy Freeman, 25 Mar. 1961, quoted in Freeman 365–366.
31. Rachel Carson to Dorothy Freeman, 1 Apr. 1962, quoted in Freeman 401. For more recent research following Carson's lead on the dangers of pesticides contaminating the food supply, see Steingraber's *Living Downstream*.
32. Rachel Carson to Dorothy Freeman, 28 Mar. 1962, quoted in Freeman 399.
33. Rachel Carson to Dorothy Freeman, 10 Apr. 1962, quoted in Freeman 404.
34. Rachel Carson to Dorothy Freeman, 20 May 1962, quoted in Freeman 405.
35. Rachel Carson to Dorothy Freeman, 25 Oct. 1962, quoted in Freeman 414.
36. Rachel Carson to Dorothy Freeman, 23 Jan. 1963, quoted in Freeman 429. For some analysis of the relationship between radiation and cancer as well as heart disease, see John Gofman's *Radiation from Medical Procedures in the Pathogenesis of Cancer and Ischemic Heart Disease*. Gofman neither denies that there is no safe dose of radiation nor advocates for its abolition in medical procedures. Rather, he believes that the rads per dose used should be dramatically reduced in all medical radiation.
37. After her appointment with Walsh, Carson added a diagnosis of angina to her list of ailments. To prevent this new complication from causing her more serious troubles, Walsh put her under a strict form of bed rest. Thus the increasing and excessive series of ailments that plagued Carson led to the additional burden of a regimented nineteenth-century rest cure. On the ways in which women writers have represented the rest cure, see Diane Price Herndl's *Figuring Feminine Illness in American Fiction and Culture*.
38. Rachel Carson to Dorothy Freeman, n.d., "Hyacinth-Time," quoted in Freeman 434.
39. Rachel Carson to Dorothy Freeman, 14 Feb. 1963, quoted in Freeman 434.
40. Rachel Carson to George Crile Jr., 17 Feb. 1963, CFP, quoted in Leopold, *A Darker*, 140–141.
41. Ibid., 142.
42. Ralph Caulk to George Crile Jr., 6 Mar. 1963, CFP, quoted in Leopold, *A Darker*, 143.
43. Rachel Carson to Dorothy Freeman, 19 Mar. 1963, quoted in Freeman 442–443. Leopold unpacked the limitations of the drug: "Tests revealed that it contained mineral oil and a form of creatine, a substance normally excreted by the body. Neither of these components has any proven anticancer activity" (Leopold, *A Darker*, 143).

44. Lear spells out that Caulk and Crile concurred that different treatments would perform much better. Caulk wanted to give Carson "short-term androgen therapy when any new areas of bone pain occurred to see if the tumor was still endocrine-sensitive. But Carson rejected this protocol since the use of male hormones had unpleasant side effects and was primarily diagnostic. She was certain her cancer was endocrine-sensitive and understood that the final treatment available to her would be either some form of adrenolectomy [removal of the adrenal glands] or a hypophysectomy, the destruction of the pituitary gland, but that was a procedure she was reluctant to submit to" (Lear, *Witness,* 446).

45. Rachel Carson to George Crile Jr., 3 Apr. 1963, CFP, quoted in Leopold, *A Darker,* 144.

46. George Crile Jr. to Rachel Carson, 5 Apr. 1963, CFP, quoted in Leopold, *A Darker,* 146.

47. Rachel Carson to Dorothy Freeman, 18 Sept. 1963, quoted in Freeman 469.

48. Rachel Carson to Dorothy Freeman, 14 Jan. 1964, quoted in Freeman 515.

49. Gofman, who was one of the scientists who worked on the Manhattan Project, has since proven that there is a link between extensive, unregulated radiation and cancer and heart disease; see his *Radiation-Induced Cancer from Low-Dose Exposure.*

50. Zillah Eisenstein updates Velsicol's investment in DDT after the laws banning its production and use in the United States went into effect in 1972, as a result of the work Carson initiated. She explains, "It remains in use as a cheap and effective control for malaria in most poor countries. As late as 1991, the u.s. exported at least 4.1 million pounds of pesticides banned or suspended from use here, including tons of DDT" (89). As Carson herself demonstrated, exporting DDT to the third world while banning it in the United States does not reduce cancer incidence and mortality rates. But it suggests that corporations manufacturing toxic chemicals continue to operate, with economic concerns overriding the ways in which exporting pesticides reproduces racism, classism, and sexism on a global scale.

51. U.S. Congress, Senate Committee on Government Operations, 62.

52. Ibid., 62.

53. Ibid., 207.

54. Carson discusses the traces of DDT found in indigenous fish near Prince of Wales Island in southeastern Alaska. No DDT had been applied to any part of the island. She cites other examples of this phenomenon in her testimony as well as in *Silent Spring.*

55. U.S. Congress, Senate Committee on Commerce, 17.

56. Ibid., 23.

57. Ibid.

58. U.S. Congress, House Committee on Government Operations.

59. Some scholarship espouses the productive potential of environmental discourse in the public sphere; see Douglas Torgerson's *The Promise of Green Politics,* and Norman Vig and Michael Kraft's *Environmental Policy.*

60. For instance, they are using an E-SCREEN bioassay, which "allows researchers to test samples to see if they act like estrogen in breast cancer cells. In addition, the Cape Study team developed and used new analytical methods to identify and measure 225 different compounds. One new method was designed to detect alkylphenols, which are breakdown products of chemicals in

some detergents and are estrogenic" (Silent Spring Institute 8). To study the changes in the Cape's environmental landscape researchers use a computer-generated mapping system called a geographic information system to learn about "water quality measurements dating as far back as 25 years, areas where pesticides were used since 1948 when DDT was first sprayed on the Cape, and land use back to 1951" (Silent Spring Institute 10). Finally, they use "sophisticated statistical analysis methods for environmental epidemiology and applied them to case-control data for the Upper Cape" (Silent Spring Institute 22). For an elaborate discussion of these scientific practices, see Ana Soto's "The E-SCREEN Assay as a Tool to Identify Estrogens" and Ruthann Rudel's "Predicting Health Effects of Exposures to Compounds with Estrogenic Activity."

61. For theories about how to implement this practice, see Devra Davis and colleagues' "Rethinking Breast Cancer Risk and the Environment."

CHAPTER 2   MEDIA MEDICAL INTERVENTIONS

1. The term *breast* was not used in the *Reader's Guide* index to periodicals until 1932, and at that time only two articles happened to be about breast cancer. Breast cancer did not have its own subcategory subject heading in the *Reader's Guide* until 1974. Prior to the events discussed in this chapter, stories in the mass media were primarily women's narratives about their experiences, and they appeared exclusively in women's magazines. In 1971 a few articles began to surface under the category *breast surgery*, although not every year. After Betty Ford's breast cancer publicity the *Reader's Guide* gave *breast* its own heading and regular subheadings like *cancer, diagnosis, surgery*, and *therapy*. According to Leslie Reagan, "One of the earliest cancer education articles appeared in 1913 in . . . [the] *Ladies' Home Journal*, a placement that foretold the importance of women's periodicals and organizations to cancer education. The article appeared thanks to the efforts of the new American Society for the Control of Cancer formed to educate the public about cancer" (1780). For further historical examinations of breast cancer publicity, see Kirsten Gardner's " 'By Women, for Women, and with Women.' "

2. For historical perspectives on the women's health movement, see Sheryl Burt Ruzek's *The Women's Health Movement* and Sandra Morgen's *Into Our Own Hands*.

3. Jane Halle Crile's breast cancer, diagnosed in 1959, often became a source of ammunition for Crile's foes, who suggested that he merely wanted revenge for his first wife's death. Jane Crile died in 1963. Even Rose Kushner initially responded to his book in this way, as I discuss in Chapter Three.

4. Campion also published excerpts from her memoir in women's magazines in the United States to share her perspective with a wider audience; see Rosamond Campion's "The Right to Choose" and "Five Years Later." Shortly after the publication of Campion's narrative, the *New York Times* picked up the story about Campion and Crile; see Judy Klemesrud's "New Voice in Debate on Breast Surgery." See Barron Lerner's *The Breast Cancer Wars* for new historical and contextual information on the relationship between Crile and Campion.

5. The difference between revealing and keeping secrets in the Ford White House, however, was not quite so clear cut. Ford and her family hid her alcoholism and drug addiction from the public for years (albeit largely because of

their denial). However, Ford did finally disclose her struggles with addiction, and obviously that legacy more profoundly affects public health in the long term than does her revelation of her breast cancer.

6. I would argue that for the Fords being public had everything to do with their membership in the Republican party. After President Nixon's Watergate scandal and subsequent resignation all politicians did not suddenly open up their lives to public scrutiny. However, the Republican party had to make up for mistakes in Nixon's administration. In this light the first lady's confession could be viewed as a way to test the effects of a particular political strategy. Although I would not take this position, it could be argued that going public with breast cancer was not entirely her decision to make. Most likely political strategists discussed its ramifications at length before concluding it would be efficacious. Examining her disclosure from this vantage point demonstrates one of several complications in her agency.

7. I mean to emphasize the Republican and "lady" qualities of Ford's rhetoric here. The first woman to be so public with breast cancer had to be white, middle-class, heterosexual, and by all appearances somewhat saintly to garner public empathy and interest in the story. These particularities of her identity also helped to establish public support, just as Rosa Parks's identity as a presentable saintly lady engendered positive publicity for the civil rights movement.

8. In her autobiography Ford often comments on her early days in Washington, D.C., when, as a regional outsider from Grand Rapids, Michigan, and to a certain extent a class outsider from a lower-middle-class family, she had to decipher the appropriate codes of dress and etiquette. Yet, ironically, when she was a little girl, her mother forced her to wear a hat and white gloves whenever she went out to play—an attempt, I would argue, to help young Betty Bloomer assimilate with upper-class girls. This contradiction seems to be best explained by the time and the context that Ford attempted to fit into as an adult. Her family offered an example of how the middle class imitates upper-class manners. I use the term *white glove* with this image in mind.

9. The year following the heightened publicity about Ford, Marvella Bayh authored a personal narrative in which she linked her struggle as a political wife enduring breast cancer to Ford's and Rockefeller's struggles. Like Ford, Bayh compared losing a breast to losing a leg, and she promised readers that losing a leg would be much worse. She reasoned that writing about breast cancer could connect her struggle to those of ordinary women who wrote letters to her and who read women's magazines. She quoted directly from letters of women with breast cancer who sought solace in a community of women who had braved the same illness.

10. Exemplary first ladies like Eleanor Roosevelt and Jacqueline Kennedy challenged norms of behavior for the wives of presidents. However, they did not call attention to their bodies in any rhetorical or visual way for a public audience. Ford modeled her political views and public persona on Roosevelt. One of Ford's lesser known political aspirations was to convince her husband to appoint a woman to the Supreme Court. The two most significant parts of Ford's legacy were that future first ladies could blur the lines between public and private and that their role as first lady widened; see Carl Anthony's *First Ladies*.

11. Two books offer historical, cultural, and political critiques of the fetishization of women's breasts: Marilyn Yalom's *A History of the Breast* and Carolyn Latteier's *Breasts*.

12. Ford locates the beginning of her mental illness at the time her husband became the minority leader of the House in 1965. However, she did not begin speaking out about it in a public forum until after she became first lady.

13. Stephen Paul Miller reads Ford in this particular style of rhetoric quite differently. He argues: "If the personal is political, it is powerless. The private and personal are no longer as revolutionary and are more acceptable. Appropriately, during the Ford years, psychoanalysis, popular and otherwise, becomes more accepted. Transactional analysis provides a way to analyze all social exchange psychoanalytically. Similarly, Betty Ford asserts her right to the public annunciation of a private life by publicizing her breast cancer and asserting that if she were younger she would try marijuana. She sets the stage for the virtual reconfiguration of American identity by glamorizing recovering from alcohol, drugs, and other 'addictions' in the mid-eighties" (344). Although I would disagree with Miller's perception that Ford's rhetoric could not be viewed as powerful, I think his explanation of the cultural and political context of Ford's utterances offers crucial insight into the ramifications of Ford's disclosures in parallel contexts.

14. Ford states later in her autobiography that as the wife of the vice president she "was already involved with the Equal Rights Amendment, and when Jerry became President, I kept pushing, trying to influence him. I used everything, including pillow talk at the end of the day, when I figured he was most tired and vulnerable." Perhaps most fascinating about Ford's description of her constant push to get the ERA passed into law was that she began the chapter about it by quoting from Shirley Temple's 1939 film *Susannah of the Mounties;* in it an American Indian boy says to Temple's character, "Squaw, keep quiet and walk behind." This quote is significant not only because of the racist image and sexist language, which upset Ford, but also because she used it to acknowledge her camaraderie with Shirley Temple Black as a breast cancer survivor: "It took the people who drafted the Equal Rights Amendment nearly forty years to catch up with Shirley, who never did walk behind. (She served her country in the UN and as Ambassador to Ghana, and even a mastectomy didn't slow her down)" (219). Despite Black's important contributions to social causes in her adult life, her progressiveness is tempered by the inescapability of the colonialist and racist representations in the films she made as a young girl. Ford's reiteration of such a representation without any commentary about its implications is not mediated by age (she was an adult); thus she gives it an even more problematic resonance.

15. Gloria Steinem was in fact an avid supporter of Ford. During Ford's tenure in the White House, Steinem printed a button that stated: "I sleep a little better every night knowing Betty Ford is sleeping with the President" (quoted in *Betty Ford: One Day at a Time*).

16. In February 1973 Shirley Temple Black wrote an article focusing on the barbaric treatment of breast cancer. Much of this personal narrative was aimed at giving women a voice and control over their bodies so that they could assert that they wanted a choice of the type of surgery to be performed—and a voice in whether there would be a surgery at all. Her rhetoric mirrors the rhetoric of a woman's right to choose in the abortion debate. Yet she also uses an apologetic tone, often directly apologizing to the medical establishment for her knowledge about breast cancer and her attempts to give advice about it. Although this pedagogical piece was groundbreaking and she received an

enormous amount of support as a result (she received fifty thousand letters, like Ford), the spotlight on breast cancer in the media was short lived. One month later the magazine carried an article by one of her doctors, George Caplan, that described the effect he hoped the disclosure of her breast cancer would have on American women.

17. Audre Lorde famously critiques the racism and heterosexism inherent in Lasser's program. For Lorde's perspective, see Chapter Four.

18. Susann's battle with breast cancer ended when she died on September 21, 1974; see Barbara Seaman's *Lovely Me*.

19. For Ripperton's story, see Bob Lucas's "Minnie Ripperton."

20. For an examination of women's embodiment located at the site of the breast, see Iris Marion Young's "Breasted Experience." Young argues that reclaiming one's breasts for oneself can be empowering because it offers sexual and maternal pleasure. However, she does not address the fears that many women have because the breast is also a site of a gendered cancer.

21. Of Ford's and Rockefeller's surgeries and the accompanying publicity, Crile states: "All of this publicity has been great for mammography and for the promotion of lesser-than-radical breast surgery, it did what I had hoped it would do. It made women examine themselves, have mammograms, and seek early treatment. Since that time, there has been a drop in the size of breast cancers that we saw and in the incidence of nodal involvement" (*Way* 395). He also reminds readers that this episode catapulted him to the center of the controversy with the AMA and ACS yet again. This time became even more fraught for Crile because by the time his second book appeared on the market, and in the wake of Ford's and Rockefeller's surgeries, Crile's second wife, Helga Sandburg Crile (daughter of poet Carl Sandburg), found a lump in her breast and had a partial mastectomy. In fact, one of *Time*'s stories covering Ford also includes photographs of Helga Crile and discusses her in the context of her husband's critique of outdated surgical practices; see "Breast Cancer: Fear and Facts." Helga Sandburg (Crile) later wrote about her experiences with breast cancer in "'Let a Joy Keep You.'"

22. Readers may find this pattern of candor suspect given that Ford used it to discuss more frivolous personal issues like her facelift in 1979. Yet it should be remembered that once she left the White House and recovered from her alcoholism and her facelift, Ford continued to actively campaign for causes like the ERA.

23. It is important to contextualize this reporter's role in the mass media. She was the first woman hired as a staff writer at *Life* magazine; she also holds the distinction of being *McCall's* first woman editor. Her opinionated positions were voiced on the CBS News radio program *Spectrum* and later on *60 Minutes* in a point-counterpoint segment featuring a man and a woman arguing about the news of the day. Moreover, if her opinions sound as though they contain a hint of backlash in response to feminism, her publishing history throws another curveball. She wrote a guidebook to women's rights that was profoundly pro-ERA and pro-choice. I would argue, however, that her objection to Ford's disclosure would still contrast with these concerns even with respect to pro-choice rhetoric because the woman's body does not figure prominently in that discourse; rather her body remains abstract.

24. Rockefeller's breast cancer was discovered on the heels of her husband's financial crisis, during which his bank accounts and books were made public.

Alexander argued that this public scrutiny was displaced onto his wife's body when her medical records were opened up in the same public fashion ("Breast").

25. For an ACS survey of this program, see Edwin Silverberg and Arthur Holleb's "Major Trends in Cancer."

26. John Gofman has researched and has proven the cumulative effects of mammography-induced cancer and heart disease in his studies; see his *Radiation-Induced Cancer from Low-Dose Exposure* and *Radiation from Medical Procedures in the Pathogenesis of Cancer and Ischemic Heart Disease.* John Bailar also publicly critiqued these screening ventures because of the high radiation doses, particularly for women in their thirties.

27. Breast cancer activists like Jane Zones explored the economic incentives for the promotion of premenopausal screening mammography: "Screening mammography for premenopausal women is the most successful example of expanding markets to increase profits. In 1972, the ACS funded 12 mammography centers in an effort to reach 60,000 women. The NCI then financed an expansion of the ACS program, and by 1975 there were 29 centers that had enrolled more than 280,000 women aged 35 to 74 years old" (138).

CHAPTER 3   ROSE KUSHNER VERSUS THE MEDICAL ESTABLISHMENT

1. Although no statisticians quantified the specific impact of Ford's and Rockefeller's disclosures on women's early detection, no one doubted their significance. However, because of the unprecedented, immediate response of women making appointments at the Breast Cancer Detection Demonstration Project, researchers attempted to quantify the later impact of First Lady Nancy Reagan's breast cancer; see Ann Nattinger and colleagues' "Effects of Nancy Reagan's Mastectomy on Choice of Surgery for Breast Cancer by U.S. Women" and Dorothy Lane, Anthony Polednak, and Mary Ann Burg's "The Impact of Media Coverage of Nancy Reagan's Experience on Breast Cancer Screening."

2. Rose Kushner to Pat Sweeting, 2 Oct. 1974, Box 7, Folder 109, Rose Kushner Collection, Schlesinger Library, Radcliffe Institute for Advanced Study (hereafter RKC); emphasis added.

3. Rose Kushner to Mrs. Nelson Rockefeller, 6 Nov. 1974, Box 7, Folder 109, RKC.

4. In this chapter I concentrate on the third edition of Kushner's text because it provides the most recent revisions to her ideas and includes the most comprehensive information about her activism; see also *Why Me?* and *Alternatives.* Leopold perceptively points out that the publishers problematically deleted the words "breast cancer" from the title of the second edition, changing it to *Why Me?* (*A Darker* 237).

5. Kushner's papers at the Schlesinger Library include several unfinished manuscripts that she attempted to publish. Her experiences reporting on war, for instance, were the genesis of three manuscripts: one book entitled *The Peacehawks,* a script entitled *Windshadow,* and a play entitled *Magyari!!!.* She also began her autobiography, *I Wasn't Raised to be a Jewish Mother,* in 1988. Because these endeavors all met dead ends while her breast cancer enabled her to find an audience, Kushner also tried to turn breast cancer into a creative subject. She coauthored a script, *A Gift of Time,* and wrote a short story,

"Hermine," about it. Her final attempt at a book, *Aerobic Sex*, argued that exercise from sex could inhibit tumor growth because it lowered lipids.

6. Rose Kushner to Jerry, 7 Oct. 1974, Box 7, Folder 109, RKC.

7. Kushner's densely written ACS brochure, *If You've Thought about Breast Cancer . . .*, provides a great deal of information for women facing breast cancer. The first edition came out in 1979. She also published articles for feminist health anthologies, such as her article "The Politics of Breast Cancer" in *Seizing Our Bodies: The Politics of Women's Health*. And she wrote articles that appeared in mainstream women's magazines—for example, "Breast Cancer: Surgery and Survival" in *Harper's Bazaar*.

8. Eleanor Turnbull used a questionnaire to prove the long-term effects of BSE for women who identified themselves as either health or nonhealth oriented. Turnbull's small sample of women (ninety health oriented; seventy nonhealth oriented) did not reveal a positive correlation between BSE and the media publicity about Ford. However, Turnbull states, "Mrs. Ford's surgical procedure and related publicity were highly influential to groups of well-educated women" (102).

9. In a letter written to Rosamond Campion's and George Crile's publisher, Kushner proposed her first breast cancer self-help book by way of a critique of their work. First, she objects to Campion's use of a pseudonym, a practice that she believes highlights and contributes to women's fears about mastectomy. Second, she believes the way that Campion refers to her doctor as the "midwest doctor" instead of naming Crile does not help women who could afford to travel to see him for the new lumpectomy surgery. Kushner wants all patients to have access to cutting-edge and accurate treatment. She culminates her criticisms by stating, "Crile cites *all* available surgeries, while Campion does not mention what I had—the modified. Again, unless I somehow misread, she leaves no alternative between the horror of the massive radical surgery and her lumpectomy" (Kushner to Medical Editor, Macmillan Publishing, 1 Aug. 1974, Box 7, Folder 108, RKC).

10. It is important to disclose that instead of chemotherapy Kushner advocates the use of tamoxifen in this article. Tamoxifen is an estrogen-blocking drug that is believed to reduce mortality in women who have estrogen receptor positive tumors. (This practice of using tamoxifen as a treatment is different from the more recent controversy over its use as a preventive substance.) She found tamoxifen to be much less toxic than the chemotherapy in wide use at the time.

11. Kushner retrieved her data from Rochelle Curtis and colleagues' study "Risk of Leukemia Associated with the First Course of Cancer Treatment."

12. Leopold is a bit more generous in her description of Kushner's writing: "The eclectic nature of her writing, its rough edges and inconclusiveness, reflect an unresolved but nevertheless clear attempt to break up the standard narrative of breast cancer experience" (*A Darker* 234).

13. At the 1979 Consensus Conference of the NCI, Kushner finally persuaded the NCI to recommend that biopsies and breast cancer surgery be separated. After this landmark victory, President Jimmy Carter appointed Kushner to a six-year term on the National Cancer Advisory Board.

14. U.S. Congress, Senate Committee on Labor and Public Welfare 11.

15. In this volume she says that, "unfortunately, the only metaphor this nonfiction

medical writer can think of is the war in Viet Nam, where the enemy could not be identified and where it was often necessary to destroy a village in order to save it" (Foreword xvi).

16. U.S. Congress, Senate Committee on Labor and Public Welfare 11. In her book, Kushner ensured that her readers would be able to apply her same tactics by including the contract she forced her surgeon to sign as a model. The only way for Kushner—or any other woman in 1974—to have control over the biopsy procedure was her surgeon signed a letter that read: "Under no circumstance is _____ or anyone else in the operating room of _____ to perform the procedure known as mastectomy (removal of either breast). I hereby release _____ and all other parties connected with the above consented-to procedure from any liability for damage sustained by me due to my refusal to consent to the performance of mastectomy (removal of either breast)" (*Alternatives* 18).

17. U.S. Congress, Senate 16.

18. In her autobiography Reagan describes her October 1987 diagnosis and her response to people like Kushner discussing it in public: "At the time of my operation, there were some people, including doctors, who thought I had taken too drastic a step in choosing the mastectomy. The director of the Breast Cancer Advisory Center was quoted in the *New York Times* as saying that my decision had 'set us back ten years' " (299). Reagan thus frames her decision to have a mastectomy—as opposed to a lumpectomy, which she was an ideal candidate for—in the rhetoric of choice.

19. Rose Kushner, interview by Anne S. Kasper, transcribed tape recording, Apr. 1983, Box 1, Folder 2, RKC, 54.

20. Ibid., 58.

21. The results of the clinical trials that began in 1976 to determine the efficacy of alternative surgeries were first made public in 1985. See Bernard Fisher and colleagues' "Five-Year Results of a Randomized Clinical Trial Comparing Total Mastectomy and Segmental Mastectomy with or without Radiation in the Treatment of Breast Cancer" and "Reanalysis and Results after 12 Years of Follow-Up in a Randomized Clinical Trial Comparing Total Mastectomy with Lumpectomy with or without Irradiation in the Treatment of Breast Cancer."

22. On this issue, also see Theresa Montini and Sheryl Ruzek's "Overturning Orthodoxy."

23. Kushner also gave testimony on several other pieces of key legislation. For example, U.S. Congress, Senate Committee on Labor and Public Welfare; U.S. Congress, House Committee on Interstate and Foreign Commerce; U.S. Congress, House Committee on Aging.

24. Montini and Ruzek quantify the relationship between heightened awareness in the general public about breast cancer and alterations in medical procedures. Specifically, they look at how texts like Kushner's books affected women's demand for choosing their own surgery and thus led eventually to eradication of the Halsted radical mastectomy. For a historical examination of the effect Kushner had on changes in medical practices, see Barron Lerner, "Inventing a Curable Disease."

25. For an analysis of the role Kushner played in altering breast cancer treatment and policy, see Montini and Ruzek.

CHAPTER 4   TOWARD TRUTH AND RECONCILIATION

1. Lorde's biographer, Alexis De Veaux, alerted me to this fact; personal communication, 30 Sept. 2002. Also see De Veaux, "Searching for Audre Lorde."

2. *The Cancer Journals* had sold approximately thirty thousand copies from its first printing with Spinster's Inc. in 1980 until 2002. Aunt Lute Books senior editor, Joan Pinkvoss, says that although this figure is not unusually high for that press, it does not reflect the number of people who have read the book because about three people read each book that gets sold. To make sure that the book remained accessible, the press promised Lorde before her death that the price would stay low. Personal communication, 4 Oct. 2002.

3. Susan Sontag most famously warns against the dangers of thinking metaphorically about cancer, urging us to consider that "illness is *not* a metaphor, and that the most truthful way of regarding illness—and the healthiest way of being ill—is one most purified of, most resistant to, metaphoric thinking" (3). Although she objects primarily to the use of, for instance, military metaphors to describe one's experience with illness, I would argue that Lorde's use of metaphors in her writing about cancer was intricately connected to her process of healing—and in many respects her healing depended on her poetic use of metaphors to describe her illness.

4. Refrain from "A Song for Many Movements," from *The Black Unicorn* by Audre Lorde. Copyright © 1978 by Audre Lorde. Used by permission of W. W. Norton & Company, Inc.

5. See, for instance, Sander Gilman's "Black Bodies, White Bodies."

6. More recently Janice Phillips studied incidence and mortality rates among black and white women to address outreach needs. Examining some of these same discrepancies in Native Hawaiian, Mexican American, Filipino, American Indian, Chinese American, Japanese American, as well as African American and Caucasian women, Sandra Underwood sees the need for community outreach in communities of color that focuses on educating women about breast self-exam, screening mammography, and clinical breast exams.

7. Diane Herndl's article on Lorde's *The Cancer Journals* ("Reconstructing") explores her own reaction to some of these issues regarding the use of a prosthesis and one's identity as a feminist.

8. Personal communication with Joan Pinkvoss, 4 Oct. 2002. For some sample syllabi and analyses of these changes, see Suzanne Poirier's "The History and Literature of Women's Health" and Marilyn McEntyre's "Touchstones."

9. Within the field of disability studies scholars have used a variety of terms to describe illness narratives. Arthur Frank calls Lorde's writing a "self-story"; Anne Hunsaker Hawkins terms it a "pathographical essay"; and G. Thomas Couser describes a subgenre called "autopathography." Although all these scholars touch on or engage with the discourses of testimony and bearing witness, I would argue that the Latin American context and history of *testimonio* best illustrate the objectives and style of Lorde's writing.

10. The ability to make such decisions about one's healthcare was a topic that Lorde researched and thought through deliberately. Part of her decision-making process about what type of surgery she would have had to do with her understanding of the relationship between traditional Western treatment and the carcinogenicity of those modalities. As she explains, "I could not choose the option of radiation and chemotherapy because I felt strongly that

everything I had read about them suggested that they were in and of themselves carcinogenic. The experimental therapies without surgery were interesting possibilities, but still unproven" (*Cancer* 32).

11. Given how candid Lorde was about most aspects of her life, especially when it
came to issues of oppression, it seems highly unlikely that Lorde knew much
about Rudolf Steiner, the founder of anthroposophic medicine. Some of
Steiner's writings are rather controversial and have been linked to early strains
of Nazism and Aryan, German nationalism. If Lorde had known about his
views on race, she likely would have found it impossible to envision a clinic
devoted to his teachings as a space of healing. DeVeaux concurs; she thinks it
unlikely that Lorde was aware of Steiner's writings or ideology. And, yet, a
couple of remarks in *A Burst of Light* make it clear that Lorde had a sense of
some oppressive threads that were unconnected to the founder of anthroposophy. For instance, she noticed while in Berlin during the summer in 1984
that "the silence about Jews is absolutely deafening, chilling" (*Burst* 58). Later,
while at the Lukas Klinik, she spoke specifically to the mood within the dogmatic, Christian healing space: "One of the cardinal rules here is that we do
not talk about our illness at mealtimes or at any social gathering, so everyone
is very polite and small-talky and banal, because of course we are all preoccupied with our bodies and the processes going on within them or else we
wouldn't be here" (*Burst* 85). Thus, even in an alternative, medical healing
center, Lorde experienced a layer of silence, which was counter to what she
believed and how she interpreted anthroposophy as well.

12. Iscador is not considered an "alternative" treatment for cancer in Europe. In
Switzerland and Germany, for instance, it is used as a traditional oncological
drug. Steiner invented the anticancer use of this mistletoe product in 1922; it
can be injected into the body by some of the same methods as those used for
chemotherapy drugs in the United States. A long-term study of the drug suggests that it can increase survival rates of cancer patients; Grossarth-Maticek et
al., "Use of Iscador."

13. See Sandra Steingraber's *Living Downstream.*

14. For an extended analysis of these intertextual connections, see Elizabeth
Alexander's "'Coming Out Blackened and Whole.'"

15. See Pat Parker's *Movement in Black,* Alicia Ostriker's *The Crack in Everything,*
Marilyn Hacker's *Winter Numbers,* Lucille Clifton's *The Terrible Stories,* Eve Sedgwick's *Tendencies,* and June Jordan's *Kissing God Goodbye* and *Affirmative Acts.*

16. Her work is excerpted in collections such as Judy Brady's *1 in 3: Women with
Cancer Confront an Epidemic,* Evelyn White's *The Black Women's Health Book,*
Hilda Raz's *Living on the Margins,* Janet Price and Margrit Shildrick's *Feminist
Theory and the Body,* and Victoria Brownworth's *Coming Out of Cancer.*

17. For an account of Love's involvement with the breast cancer movement, see
Karin Stabiner's *To Dance with the Devil.*

18. The center is also named for Michael Callen, a gay man who died of AIDS in
1993; see Ian Fisher's "Health Care for Lesbians Gets a Sharper Focus." In Los
Angeles, at the L.A. Gay and Lesbian Community Services Center a healthcare facility is called The Audre Lorde Lesbian Health Clinic.

19. Two studies historicize Lorde's role in the breast cancer movement: Ulrike
Boehmer's *The Personal and the Political* and Bonnie Spanier's "'Your Silence
Will Not Protect You.'"

20. For material about the founding of Avery's organization, see her "Breathing

Life into Ourselves." For current projects that the NBWHP is working on, view their website: www.blackwomenshealth.org.

21. Mary Anglin suggests that such an implicit link connects the writings of women like Kushner and Lorde to the political changes that grew out of the ideas these women disseminated in the public sphere. See Anglin's "Working from the Inside Out."

22. For instance, Marcia Bayne-Smith points out that the health status of people of color in all medical contexts is based on political and economic inequities. She cites four reasons to support this claim: "First, gaining access to high-quality health care is expensive because it is the most lucrative service industry in the United States. . . . Second, because the health care industry is such a profitable institution the entire system is extremely politicized. . . . Third, when heath care services are being developed for the poor, rarely are the very people who will become the consumers of the services ever present at those planning sessions or high level negotiations. . . . Fourth, only occasionally do the poor manage to become sufficiently organized politically to make their presence felt" (12). But I would argue that narratives like Lorde's can be a crucial method of having consumer voices heard by those organizing and maintaining the healthcare system.

23. For some of these studies, see Lisa Newman et al.'s "African-American Ethnicity, Socioeconomic Status, and Breast Cancer Survival"; Balius Walker, Larry Figgs, and Sheila Zahm's "Differences in Cancer Incidence, Mortality, and Survival between African Americans and Whites"; Nancy Krieger's "Social Class and Black/White Crossover in the Age-Specific Incidence of Breast Cancer"; Nancy Krieger et al.'s "Breast Cancer and Serum Organochlorines" and "Social Class, Race/Ethnicity, and Incidence of Breast, Cervix, Colon, Lung, and Prostate Cancer among Asian, Black, Hispanic, and White Residents of the San Francisco Bay Area, 1988–92"; and Jill Moormier's "Breast Cancer in Black Women."

CONCLUSION: TAKING ACTION

1. A copy of this report can be viewed at www.unfpa.org.

2. For more detailed material on Asian migration and breast cancer incidence rates, see Michelle Pineda and colleagues' "Asian Breast Cancer Survival in the U.S."

3. Eisenstein documents some of her conversations with women in countries like Ghana and India. For instance, she observes that, in Delhi's Cancer Sahyog, in "an emotional support group for people living with cancer and their families very many of the women who had had mastectomies refused to leave their homes. . . . If only good prostheses could be made available to them, their lives would greatly improve. Prostheses in india are made of rubber, are too lightweight and flimsy, and most women even if they can afford them won't wear them" (163). It is hard to determine whether such a response is widespread. But many of Eisenstein's conclusions suggest, as one would expect, that different cultural norms govern the way women view breast cancer.

4. Some of the websites make selling pink-ribbon products a priority. To a certain extent this is a fundraising opportunity for nonprofit organizations, and, at least initially, this was a method of raising awareness about the disease. More

recently, however, the consumption of pink-ribbon products has become excessive and undermines the political work of many breast cancer activists. See Ellen Leopold's "Shopping for the Cure."

5. For a history of Mary-Claire King's search for BRCA1, see Karin Stabiner's *To Dance with the Devil.*

6. If the risk were absolute, a woman who took HRT would necessarily find herself with breast cancer; relative risk refers to the likelihood that a woman would find herself with the disease.

7. On this study, see Barbara Brenner's "Sister Support" and Sandra Steingraber's "The Environmental Link to Breast Cancer."

8. See Marilie Gammon and colleagues' "Environmental Toxins and Breast Cancer on Long Island I" and "Environmental Toxins and Breast Cancer on Long Island II."

References

Aitken, Malcolm. "Gulf War Leaves Legacy of Cancer." *British Medical Journal* 319 (1999): 401.

Alexander, Elizabeth. "'Can You Be BLACK and Look at This?': Reading the Rodney King Video(s)." *The Black Public Sphere*. Ed. Black Public Sphere Collective. Chicago: University of Chicago Press, 1995. 81–98.

———. "'Coming Out Blackened and Whole': Fragmentation and Reintegration in Audre Lorde's *Zami* and *The Cancer Journals*." *American Literary History* 6.4 (1994): 695–715.

Alexander, Shana. "Breast Cancer and News Overkill." *Newsweek* 9 Dec. 1974: 122.

al-Radi, Nuha. *Baghdad Diaries: A Woman's Chronicle of War and Exile*. New York: Vintage Books, 2003.

Angelo, Bonnie. "The Relentless Ordeal of Political Wives." *Time* 7 Oct. 1974: 15–22.

Anglin, Mary K. "Working from the Inside Out: Implications of Breast Cancer Activism for Biomedical Policies and Practices." *Social Science Medicine* 44 (1997): 1403–1415.

Anthony, Carl Sferrazza. *First Ladies*. Vol. 2, *1961–1990: The Saga of the Presidents' Wives and Their Power*. New York: Quill, 1993.

Austin, Mary. *Earth Horizon: Autobiography*. New York: Literary Guild, 1932.

Avery, Byllye Y. "Breathing Life into Ourselves: The Evolution of the National Black Women's Health Project." *The Black Women's Health Book: Speaking for Ourselves*. Ed. Evelyn C. White. Seattle: Seal Press, 1990. 4–10.

Bailar, John C., III. "Mammography: A Contrary View." *Annals of Internal Medicine* 84 (1976): 77–84.

Baker, Larry H. "Breast Cancer Detection Demonstration Project: Five-Year Summary Report." *CA-A Cancer Journal for Clinicians* 32.4 (1982): 194–225.

Bassett, Mary T., and Nancy Krieger. "Social Class and Black-White Differences in Breast Cancer Survival." *American Journal of Public Health* 76 (1986): 1400–1403.

Batt, Sharon. *Patient No More: The Politics of Breast Cancer*. Charlottetown, P.E.I., Canada: gynergy books, 1994.

Bayh, Marvella. "Betty, Happy . . . and Me." *Ladies' Home Journal* Jan. 1975: 63+.

Bayne-Smith, Marcia, ed. *Race, Gender, and Health*. Thousand Oaks, Calif.: Sage, 1996.

Betty Ford: One Day at a Time. New York: A&E Biography, 1996.

"Betty Ford's Operation." *Newsweek* 7 Oct. 1974: 30–33.

Black, Shirley Temple. "Don't Sit Home and Be Afraid." *McCall's* Feb. 1973: 82+.

Blair, Carole. "Contemporary U.S. Memorial Sites as Exemplars of Rhetoric's Materiality." *Rhetorical Bodies*. Ed. Jack Selzer and Sharon Crowley. Madison: University of Wisconsin Press, 1999. 16–57.

Boehmer, Ulrike. *The Personal and the Political: Women's Activism in Response to the Breast Cancer and AIDS Epidemics*. Albany: State University of New York Press, 2000.

Bosso, Christopher J. *Pesticides and Politics: The Life Cycle of a Public Issue*. Pittsburgh: University of Pittsburgh Press, 1987.

Boston Women's Health Book Collective. *Our Bodies, Ourselves*. New York: Simon & Schuster, 1971.

Boyer, Paul. *By the Bomb's Early Light: American Thought and Culture at the Dawn of the Atomic Age*. 1985. Chapel Hill: University of North Carolina Press, 1994.

Brady, Judy, ed. *1 in 3: Women with Cancer Confront an Epidemic*. Pittsburgh: Cleis Press, 1991.

"Breast Cancer: Fear and Facts." *Time* 4 Nov. 1974: 107–110.

"Breast Cancer Study Finds Radical Surgery Has No Advantage over Simple Mastectomy." *New York Times* 30 Sept. 1974: 26.

Brenner, Barbara A. "From the Executive Director: Educate, Agitate, Organize— Now!" *Breast Cancer Action Newsletter* 49 (1998) <www.bcaction.org/Pages/ SearchablePages/ 1998newsletters /Newsletter049A.html>.

———. "Lessons from Long Island." *Breast Cancer Action Newsletter* 74 (2002): 2.

———. "Sister Support: Women Create a Breast Cancer Movement." *Breast Cancer: Society Shapes an Epidemic*. Ed. Anne S. Kasper and Susan J. Ferguson. New York: St. Martin's Press, 2000. 325–353.

———. "Waging War, Making Connections." *Breast Cancer Action Newsletter* 78 (2003): 2.

Brody, Jane E. "Fast Action Vital in Cancer Cases." *New York Times* 29 Sept. 1974: 23+.

———. "Inquiries Soaring on Breast Cancer." *New York Times* 6 Oct. 1974: 21+.

Brooks, Paul. *The House of Life: Rachel Carson at Work*. Boston: Houghton Mifflin, 1972.

Brownworth, Victoria A., ed. *Coming Out of Cancer: Writings from the Lesbian Cancer Epidemic*. Seattle: Seal Press, 2000.

Burney, Frances. *The Journals and Letters of Fanny Burney*. Ed. Joyce Hemlow. Vol. 6. Oxford: Clarendon Press, 1975.

Campion, Rosamond [pseud. of Babette Rosamond]. "Five Years Later." *McCall's* June 1976: 113+.

———. *The Invisible Worm*. New York: Macmillan, 1972.

———. "The Right to Choose." *McCall's* Feb. 1972: 64+.

Caplan, Gerald. "An Outpouring of Love for Shirley Temple Black." *McCall's* Mar. 1973: 48–54.

Carson, Rachel. *Lost Woods: The Discovered Writing of Rachel Carson*. Ed. Linda Lear. Boston: Beacon Press, 1998.

———. *The Sea around Us*. Rev. ed. New York: Oxford University Press, 1961.

———. *Silent Spring*. Boston: Houghton Mifflin, 1962.

Clifton, Lucille. *The Terrible Stories*. Brockport, N.Y.: BOA Editions, 1996.

Clinton, Hillary Rodham. "Remembering Virginia." *Ladies' Home Journal* May 1998: 114–115.

"A Confirmation Fight Shapes Up." *Time* 28 Oct. 1974: 18–20.

Cook, Karin. *What Girls Learn*. New York: Pantheon Books, 1997.

Cooke, Cynthia W., and Susan Dworkin. *The Ms. Guide to a Woman's Health*. New York: Doubleday, 1979.

Cottam, Clarence, and Elmer Higgins. "DDT and Its Effect on Fish and Wildlife." *Journal of Economic Entomology* 39 (1946): 44–52.

Couser, G. Thomas. *Recovering Bodies: Illness, Disability, and Life Writing*. Madison: University of Wisconsin Press, 1997.

Crile, George, Jr. "Breast Cancer: A Patient's Bill of Rights." *Ms*. Sept. 1973: 66+.

———. *Cancer and Common Sense*. New York: Viking Press, 1955.

———. "A Plea against Blind Fear of Cancer." *Life* 31 Oct. 1955: 140.

———. *The Way It Was: Sex, Surgery, Treasure, and Travel, 1907–1987*. Kent, Ohio: Kent State University Press, 1992.

———. *What Women Should Know about the Breast Cancer Controversy*. New York: Macmillan, 1973.

Curtis, Rochelle E., et al. "Risk of Leukemia Associated with the First Course of Cancer Treatment: An Analysis of the Surveillance, Epidemiology, and End Results Program Experience." *Journal of the National Cancer Institute* 72 (1984): 531–544.

Dally, Ann. *Women under the Knife: A History of Surgery*. New York: Routledge, 1992.

Daniel, Pete. "A Rogue Bureaucracy: The USDA Fire Ant Campaign of the Late 1950s." *Agricultural History* 64 (1990): 99–103.

Davis, Devra Lee, et al. "Rethinking Breast Cancer Risk and the Environment: The Case for the Precautionary Principle." *Environmental Health Perspectives* 106 (1998): 523–529.

Degen, Clara, and Kathleen Wilkinson. "Town Meeting Inspires Activism." *Breast Cancer Action Newsletter* 51 (1999) <www.bcaction.org/Pages/SearchablePages/1998newsletters/Newsletter051A.html>.

Delgado, Jane, ed. *¡Salud!: A Latina's Guide to Total Health—Body, Mind, and Spirit*. New York: Harper Perennial, 1997.

de Moulin, Daniel. *A Short History of Breast Cancer*. Boston: Martinus Nijhoff, 1983.

De Veaux, Alexis. "Searching for Audre Lorde." *Callaloo* 23. 1 (2000): 64–67.

Dickersin, Kay, and Lauren Schnaper. "Reinventing Medical Research." *Man-Made Medicine: Women's Health, Public Policy, and Reform*. Ed. Kary L. Moss. Durham: Duke University Press, 1996. 57–75.

Dreifus, Claudia, ed. *Seizing Our Bodies: The Politics of Women's Health*. New York: Vintage Books, 1978.

Dunlap, Thomas R. *DDT: Scientists, Citizens, and Public Policy*. Princeton: Princeton University Press, 1981.

Edelman, Hope. *Letters from Motherless Daughters: Words of Courage, Grief, and Healing*. New York: Delta, 1996.

———. *Motherless Daughters: The Legacy of Loss*. New York: Delta, 1994.

Eisenstein, Zillah. *Manmade Breast Cancers*. Ithaca: Cornell University Press, 2001.

Epstein, Julia. *The Iron Pen: Frances Burney and the Politics of Women's Writing*. Madison: University of Wisconsin Press, 1989.

Epstein, Samuel S. *The Politics of Cancer Revisited*. 1978. Rpt., 2 vols. in 1. Fremont Center, N.Y.: East Ridge Press, 1998.

Faderman, Lillian. *Surpassing the Love of Men: Romantic Friendship and Love between Women from the Renaissance to the Present.* New York: Morrow, 1981.

Fee, Elizabeth, ed. *The Politics of Sex in Medicine.* Farmingdale, N.Y.: Baywood, 1983.

Felski, Rita. *Beyond Feminist Aesthetics: Feminist Literature and Social Change.* Cambridge: Harvard University Press, 1989.

Fisher, Bernard, et al. "Five-Year Results of a Randomized Clinical Trial Comparing Total Mastectomy and Segmental Mastectomy with or without Radiation in the Treatment of Breast Cancer." *New England Journal of Medicine* 312 (1985): 665–673.

————. "Reanalysis and Results after 12 Years of Follow-Up in a Randomized Clinical Trial Comparing Total Mastectomy with Lumpectomy with or without Irradiation in the Treatment of Breast Cancer." *New England Journal of Medicine* 333 (1995): 1456–1461.

Fisher, Ian. "Health Care for Lesbians Gets a Sharper Focus." *New York Times* 21 June 1998: 27.

Flaws, Jodi A., Craig J. Newschaffer, and Trudy L. Bush. "Breast Cancer Mortality in Black and White Women: A Historical Perspective by Menopausal Status." *Journal of Women's Health* 7 (1998): 1007–1015.

Fletcher, Suzanne W., and Graham A. Colditz. "Failure of Estrogen Plus Progestin Therapy for Prevention." *Journal of the American Medical Association* 288 (2002): 366–369.

Ford, Betty, with Chris Chase. *The Times of My Life.* New York: Ballantine, 1978.

Frank, Arthur W. *The Wounded Storyteller: Body, Illness, and Ethics.* Chicago: University of Chicago Press, 1995.

Fraser, Nancy. "Rethinking the Public Sphere: A Contribution to the Critique of Actually Existing Democracy." *The Phantom Public Sphere.* Ed. Bruce Robbins. Minneapolis: University of Minnesota Press, 1993. 1–32.

————. "Sex, Lies, and the Public Sphere: Reflections on the Confirmation of Clarence Thomas." *Feminism: The Public and the Private.* Ed. Joan B. Landes. New York: Oxford University Press, 1998. 314–337.

Freeman, Martha, ed. *Always, Rachel: The Letters of Rachel Carson and Dorothy Freeman, 1952–1964.* Boston: Beacon Press, 1995.

Gammon, Marilie D., et al. "Environmental Toxins and Breast Cancer on Long Island I: Polycyclic Aromatic Hydrocarbon DNA Adducts." *Cancer Epidemiology, Biomarkers & Prevention* 11 (2002): 677–685.

————. "Environmental Toxins and Breast Cancer on Long Island II: Organochlorine Compound Levels in Blood." *Cancer Epidemiology, Biomarkers & Prevention* 11 (2002): 686–697.

Gardner, Kirsten E. "'By Women, for Women, and with Women': A History of Female Cancer Efforts in the United States, 1913–1970s." Diss., University of Cincinnati, 1999.

Gibbons-Knopf, Jane. "The War inside My Body." *Unbearable Uncertainty: The Fear of Breast Cancer Recurrence, an Anthology.* Ed. Amy Bowes, Terry S. Gingras, Beth A. Kaplowitt, and Anne Perkins. Northampton, Mass.: Pioneer Valley Breast Cancer Network, 2000. 117–129.

Gilman, Charlotte Perkins. *The Living of Charlotte Perkins Gilman.* 1935. Madison: University of Wisconsin Press, 1990.

Gilman, Sander L. "Black Bodies, White Bodies: Toward an Iconography of Female

Sexuality in Late Nineteenth-Century Art, Medicine, and Literature." *"Race," Writing, and Difference*. Ed. Henry Louis Gates Jr. Chicago: University of Chicago Press, 1985. 223–261.

Gofman, John W. *Radiation from Medical Procedures in the Pathogenesis of Cancer and Ischemic Heart Disease: Dose-Response Studies with Physicians per 100,000 Population*. Ed. Egan O'Connor. San Francisco: Committee for Nuclear Responsibility, 1999.

———. *Radiation-Induced Cancer from Low-Dose Exposure: An Independent Analysis*. San Francisco: Committee for Nuclear Responsibility, 1990.

Graham, Frank, Jr. *Since Silent Spring*. Boston: Houghton Mifflin, 1970.

Grossarth-Maticek, Ronald, et al. "Use of Iscador, an Extract of European Mistletoe (*Viscum Album*), in Cancer Treatment: Prospective Nonrandomized and Randomized Matched-Pair Studies Nested within a Cohort Study." *Alternative Therapies* 7.3 (2001): 57–75.

Grosz, Elizabeth. *Space, Time, and Perversion*. New York: Routledge, 1995.

Habermas, Jürgen. *The Structural Transformation of the Public Sphere*. Trans. Thomas Burger. Cambridge: MIT Press, 1991.

Hacker, Marilyn. *Winter Numbers: Poems*. New York: Norton, 1994.

Halsted, William Stewart. "The Results of Operations for the Cure of Cancer of the Breast Performed at the Johns Hopkins Hospital from June 1889 to January 1894." *Surgical Papers, 1852–1922*. 2nd ed. Vol. 2. Baltimore: Johns Hopkins University Press, 1952. 3–50.

"Happy's Brush with Cancer." *Newsweek* 28 Oct. 1974: 29.

Harrison, Andrew, and W. G. MacCallum. *William Stewart Halsted*. Baltimore: Johns Hopkins University Press, 1930.

Hartmann, Lynn C., et al. "Efficacy of Bilateral Prophylactic Mastectomy in Women with a Family History of Breast Cancer." *New England Journal of Medicine* 340 (1999): 77–84.

"A Hectic Week for Breast Cancer Researchers." *Medical World News* 25 Oct. 1974: 19–22.

Herndl, Diane Price. *Figuring Feminine Illness in American Fiction and Culture, 1840–1940*. Chapel Hill: University of North Carolina Press, 1993.

———. "Reconstructing the Posthuman Feminist Body Twenty Years after Audre Lorde's *Cancer Journals*." *Disability Studies: Enabling the Humanities*. Ed. Sharon L. Snyder, Brenda Jo Brueggemann, and Rosemarie Garland-Thomsaon. New York: Modern Language Association, 2002. 144–155.

Hogeland, Lisa Maria. *Feminism and Its Fictions: The Consciousness-Raising Novel and the Women's Liberation Movement*. Philadelphia: University of Pennsylvania Press, 1998.

Hotchkiss, Neil, and Richard H. Pough. "Effect on Forest Birds of DDT Used for Gypsy Moth Control in Pennsylvania." *Journal of Wildlife Management* 10 (1946): 202–207.

Hunsaker Hawkins, Anne. *Reconstructing Illness: Studies in Pathography*. 2nd ed. West Lafayette: Purdue University Press, 1999.

Hunter, Marjorie. "Ford's Wife Undergoes Breast Cancer Surgery." *New York Times* 29 Sept. 1974: 1+.

Jacobs, Harriet A. *Incidents in the Life of a Slave Girl Written by Herself*. 1861. Ed. Jean Fagan Yellin. Cambridge: Harvard University Press, 1987.

James, Alice. *Alice James: Her Brothers, Her Journal.* Ed. Anna Robeson Burr. New York: Dodd, Mead, 1934.

Jemal, Ahmedin, et al. "Cancer Statistics, 2002." *CA: Cancer Journal for Clinicians* 52 (2002): 23–47.

Johnson, Sharon. "My Side: Rose Kushner." *Working Woman* 8 (May 1983): 160–161.

Johnson-Tekahoinwake, E. Pauline. *Flint and Feather: The Complete Poems of E. Pauline Johnson (Tekahionwake).* 1912. Toronto: Musson Book Company, 1967.

Jordan, June. *Affirmative Acts: Political Essays.* New York: Anchor Books, 1998.

———. *Kissing God Goodbye: Poems, 1991–1997.* New York: Anchor Books, 1998.

Kahane, Deborah Hobler. *No Less a Woman: Ten Women Shatter the Myths about Breast Cancer.* New York: Fireside, 1990.

Kaufert, Patricia A. "Women and the Debate over Mammography: An Economic, Political, and Moral History." *Gender and Health: An International Perspective.* Ed. Carolyn F. Sargent and Caroline B. Brettell. Upper Saddle River, N.J.: Prentice Hall, 1996. 167–186.

Klemesrud, Judy. "After Breast Cancer Operations, a Difficult Emotional Adjustment." *New York Times* 1 Oct. 1974: 46+.

———. "New Voice in Debate on Breast Surgery." *New York Times* 12 Dec. 1972: 56.

Koedt, Anne, Ellen Levine, and Anita Rapone, eds. *Radical Feminism.* New York: Quadrangle, 1973.

Krause, Arthur S., and Abraham Oppenheim. "Trend of Mortality from Cancer of the Breast." *Journal of the American Medical Association* 194 (1965): 201–202.

Krieger, Nancy. "Social Class and Black/White Crossover in the Age-Specific Incidence of Breast Cancer." *American Journal of Epidemiology* 131 (1990): 804–814.

Krieger, Nancy, and Elizabeth Fee. "Man-Made Medicine and Women's Health: The Biopolitics of Sex/Gender and Race/Ethnicity." *Man-Made Medicine: Women's Health, Public Policy, and Reform.* Ed. Kary L. Moss. Durham: Duke University Press, 1996. 15–35.

Krieger, Nancy, et al. "Breast Cancer and Serum Organochlorines: A Prospective Study among White, Black, and Asian Women." *Journal of the National Cancer Institute* 86 (1994): 589–599.

———. "Social Class, Race/Ethnicity, and Incidence of Breast, Cervix, Colon, Lung, and Prostate Cancer among Asian, Black, Hispanic, and White Residents of the San Francisco Bay Area, 1988–92." *Cancer Causes and Control* 10 (1999): 525–537.

Kushner, Rose. *Alternatives: New Developments in the War on Breast Cancer.* 3rd ed. New York: Warner Books, 1984.

———. *Breast Cancer: A Personal History and an Investigative Report.* 1975. 3rd ed. New York: Harcourt Brace Jovanovich, 1984.

———. "Breast Cancer Surgery." *Washington Post* 6 Oct. 1974: C2.

———. "Breast Cancer Surgery and Survival." *Harper's Bazaar* Sept. 1976: 146–147.

———. Foreword. *Her Soul Beneath the Bone: Women's Poetry on Breast Cancer.* Ed. Leatrice H. Lifshitz. Urbana: University of Illinois Press, 1988. xiii–xxii.

————. *If You've Thought about Breast Cancer . . .* 1979. Rpt. Ed. Harvey D. Kushner. Kensington, Md.: Rose Kushner Breast Cancer Advisory Center, 1994.

————. "Is Aggressive Adjuvant Chemotherapy the Halsted Radical of the '80s?" *CA: A Cancer Journal for Clinicians* 34 (1984): 344–351.

————. "The Politics of Breast Cancer." *Seizing Our Bodies: The Politics of Women's Health.* Ed. Claudia Dreifus. New York: Vintage Books, 1978. 186–194.

————. *Why Me?* 2nd ed. of *Breast Cancer.* Philadelphia: Saunders, 1982.

Lane, Dorothy S., Anthony P. Polednak, and Mary Ann Burg. "The Impact of Media Coverage of Nancy Reagan's Experience on Breast Cancer Screening." *American Journal of Public Health* 79 (1989): 1551–1552.

Langreth, Robert. "Study Backs the Removal of Breasts in the Fight to Lower Risks of Cancer." *Wall Street Journal* 14 Jan. 1999: 1.

Latteier, Carolyn. *Breasts: The Woman's Perspective on an American Obsession.* New York: Harrington Park, 1998.

Lear, Linda J. "Bombshell in Beltsville: The USDA and the Challenge of 'Silent Spring.'" *Agricultural History* 66 (1992): 151–170.

————. *Rachel Carson: [Witness] for Nature.* New York: Henry Holt, 1997.

————. "Rachel Carson's *Silent Spring.*" *Environmental History Review* 17 (1993): 23–48.

Leopold, Ellen. *A Darker Ribbon: Breast Cancer, Women, and Their Doctors in the Twentieth Century.* Boston: Beacon Press, 1999.

————. "Shopping for the Cure." *Breast Cancer Action Newsletter* 63 (2001): 1+.

Lerner, Barron H. *The [Breast Cancer] Wars: Hope, Fear, and the Pursuit of a Cure in Twentieth-Century America.* New York: Oxford University Press, 2001.

————. "Inventing a Curable Disease: Historical Perspectives on Breast Cancer." *Breast Cancer: Society Shapes an Epidemic.* Ed. Anne S. Kasper and Susan J. Ferguson. New York: St. Martin's Press, 2000. 25–50.

Lorde, Audre. *A Burst of Light.* Ithaca: Firebrand Press, 1988.

————. *The Cancer Journals.* 1980. Spec. ed. San Francisco: Aunt Lute Books, 1997.

————. *Sister Outsider.* Freedom, Calif.: Crossing Press, 1984.

————. *Zami: A New Spelling of My Name.* Freedom, Calif.: Crossing Press, 1982.

Love, Susan, with Karen Lindsey. *Dr. Susan Love's Breast Book,* 2nd ed. Reading, Mass.: Perseus Books, 1995.

Lucas, Bob. "Minnie Ripperton: Singing Star Discusses Her Recent Surgery for Breast Cancer." *Ebony* Dec. 1976: 33–42.

Lutts, Ralph H. "Chemical Fallout: Rachel Carson's *Silent Spring,* Radioactive Fallout, and the Environmental Movement." *Environmental Review* 9 (1985): 210–225

"Mammography 1982: A Statement of the American Cancer Society." *CA-A: Cancer Journal for Clinicians* 32.4 (1982): 226–231.

Marco, Gino J., Robert M. Hollingworth, and William Durham, eds. *Silent Spring Revisited.* Washington: American Chemical Society, 1987.

McCauley, Linda A., et al. "Illness Experience of Gulf War Veterans Possibly Exposed to Chemical Warfare Agents." *American Journal of Preventive Medicine* 23 (2003): 200–206.

McDowell, Deborah E. "Recovery Missions: Imaging the Body Ideals." *Recovering*

the Black Female Body: Self-Representations by African American Women. Ed.
Michael Bennett and Vanessa D. Dickerson. New Brunswick: Rutgers University Press, 2001. 296–317.

McEntyre, Marilyn Chandler. "Touchstones: A Brief Survey of Some Standard Works." *Teaching Literature and Medicine*. Ed. Anne Hunsaker Hawkins and Marilyn Chandler McEntyre. New York: Modern Language Association, 2000. 187–199.

McKay, Nellie Y. "The Narrative Self: Race, Politics, and Culture in Black American Women's Autobiography." *Women, Autobiography, Theory: A Reader*. Ed. Sidonie Smith and Julia Watson. Madison: University of Wisconsin Press, 1998. 96–107.

McWhorter, William P., and William J. Mayer. "Black/White Differences in Type of Initial Breast Cancer Treatment and Implications for Survival." *American Journal of Public Health* 77 (1987): 1515–1517.

Medhurst, Martin J., et al., eds. *Cold War Rhetoric: Strategy, Metaphor, and Ideology*. Westport, Conn.: Greenwood Press, 1990.

Miller, Stephen Paul. *The Seventies Now: Culture as Surveillance*. Durham: Duke University Press, 1999.

Montague, Peter. "Radiation Causes Breast Cancer." *Rachel's Environment & Health Weekly* 443 (25 May 1995): 3.

Montini, Theresa, and Sheryl Ruzek. "Overturning Orthodoxy: The Emergence of Breast Cancer Treatment Policy." *Research in the Sociology of Health Care: A Research Annual*. Ed. Dorothy C. Wertz. Vol. 8. Greenwich, Conn.: JAI Press, 1989. 3–32.

Moormeier, Jill. "Breast Cancer in Black Women." *Annals of Internal Medicine* 124 (1996): 897–905.

Morgen, Sandra. *Into Our Own Hands: The Women's Health Movement in the United States, 1969–1990*. New Brunswick: Rutgers University Press, 2002.

Nattinger, Ann, et al. "Effects of Nancy Reagan's Mastectomy on Choice of Surgery for Breast Cancer by U.S. Women." *Journal of the American Medical Association* 279 (1988): 762–766.

Nelkin, Dorothy, and Sander L. Gilman. "Placing Blame for Devastating Disease." *Social Research* 55 (1988): 361–378.

Newman, Lisa A., et al. "African-American Ethnicity, Socioeconomic Status, and Breast Cancer Survival: A Meta-Analysis of 14 Studies Involving over 10,000 African-American and 40,000 White American Patients with Carcinoma of the Breast." *Cancer* 94.11 (2002): 2844–2854.

Obaid, Thoraya Ahmed. *UNFPA State of World Population 2002: People, Poverty, and Possibilities*. New York: United Nations Population Fund, 2002.

Olson, James S. *Bathsheba's Breast: Women, Cancer, and History*. Baltimore: Johns Hopkins University Press, 2002.

Ostriker, Alicia Suskin. *The Crack in Everything*. Pittsburgh: University of Pittsburgh Press, 1996.

Parker, Pat. *Movement in Black*. 1978. Expanded ed. Ithaca: Firebrand Books, 1999.

Parkin, D. Max, et al. "Global Cancer Statistics." *CA—A Cancer Journal for Clinicians* 49 (1999): 33–64.

Patterson, James T. *The Dread Disease: Cancer and Modern American Culture*. Cambridge: Harvard University Press, 1987.

Phillips, Janice Mitchell. "Breast Cancer and African American Women." *Contemporary Issues in Breast Cancer*. Ed. Karen Hassey Dow. Boston: Jones & Bartlett, 1996. 219–228.

Pineda, Michelle D., et al. "Asian Breast Cancer Survival in the U.S.: A Comparison between Asian Immigrants, U.S.-Born Asian Americans, and Caucasians." *International Journal of Epidemiology* 30 (2001): 976–982.

Poirier, Suzanne. "The History and Literature of Women's Health." *Teaching Literature and Medicine*. Ed. Anne Hunsaker Hawkins and Marilyn Chandler McEntyre. New York: Modern Language Association, 2000. 65–76.

Price, Janet, and Margrit Shildrick, eds. *Feminist Theory and the Body: A Reader*. New York: Routledge, 1999.

Probyn, Elspeth. "This Body Which Is Not One: Speaking an Embodied Self." *Hypatia* 6 (1991): 111–124.

Proctor, Robert N. *Cancer Wars: How Politics Shapes What We Know and Don't Know about Cancer*. New York: Basic Books, 1995.

Radner, Gilda. *It's Always Something*. New York: Simon & Schuster, 1989.

Raffensperger, Carolyn. "Wingspread Conference on the Precautionary Principle." (Jan. 1998). Science and Environmental Health Network. Accessed 1 Jan. 2004. <www.sehn.org/wing.html>

Raz, Hilda, ed. *Living on the Margins: Women Writers on Breast Cancer*. New York: Persea Books, 1999.

Reagan, Leslie J. "Engendering the Dread Disease: Women, Men, and Cancer." *American Journal of Public Health* 87 (1997): 1779–1787.

Reagan, Nancy, with William Novak. *My Turn: The Memoirs of Nancy Reagan*. New York: Dell, 1989.

Rockefeller, Margaretta "Happy," as told to Eleanor Harris. "If It Should Happen to You." *Reader's Digest* May 1976: 131–134.

Rowell, Charles H. "Above the Wind: An Interview with Audre Lorde." *Callaloo* 23.1 (2000): 52–63.

Rudel, Ruthann. "Predicting Health Effects of Exposures to Compounds with Estrogenic Activity: Methodological Issues." *Environmental Health Perspectives* 105, supp. 3 (1997): 655–663.

Ruzek, Sheryl Burt. *The Women's Health Movement: Feminist Alternatives to Medical Control*. New York: Praeger, 1978.

Ruzek, Sheryl Burt, and Julie Becker. "The Women's Health Movement in the United States: From Grass-Roots Activism to Professional Agendas." *Journal of the American Medical Women's Association* 54 (1999): 4–8.

Sandburg [Crile], Helga. "'Let a Joy Keep You.'" *McCall's* Nov. 1974: 63+.

Schain, Wendy S. "Physician-Patient Communication about Breast Cancer." *Surgical Clinics of North America* 70 (1990): 917–936.

Seaman, Barbara. *Lovely Me: The Life of Jacqueline Susann*. 1987. New York: Seven Stories, 1996.

Sedgwick, Eve Kosofsky. *Tendencies*. Durham: Duke University Press, 1993.

Sherman, Janette. *Life's Delicate Balance: Guide to Causes and Prevention of Breast Cancer*. New York: Taylor & Francis, 2000.

Silent Spring Institute. *The Cape Cod Breast Cancer and Environment Study: Results of the First Three Years of Study*. Newton, Mass.: Silent Spring Institute, 1998.

Silverberg, Edwin, and Arthur Holleb. "Major Trends in Cancer: 25 Year Survey." *CA—A Cancer Journal for Clinicians* 25 (1975): 2–7.

Smart, Charles et al. "Twenty-Year Follow Up of the Breast Cancers Diagnosed during the Breast Cancer Detection Demonstration Project." *CA—A Cancer Journal for Clinicians* 47 (1997): 134–149.

Smith, Sidonie. *Subjectivity, Identity, and the Body: Women's Autobiographical Practices in the Twentieth Century.* Bloomington: Indiana University Press, 1993.

Smith-Rosenberg, Carroll. *Disorderly Conduct: Visions of Gender in Victorian America.* New York: Knopf, 1985.

Sontag, Susan. *Illness as Metaphor and AIDS and Its Metaphors.* New York: Anchor Books, 1988.

Soto, Ana M., et al. "The E-SCREEN Assay as a Tool to Identify Estrogens: An Update on Estrogenic Environmental Pollutants." *Environmental Health Perspectives* 103, supp. 7 (1995): 113–122.

Spanier, Bonnie. "'Your Silence Will Not Protect You': Feminist Science Studies, Breast Cancer, and Activism." *Feminist Science Studies: A New Generation.* Ed. Maralee Mayberry, Banu Subramaniam, and Lisa H. Weasel. New York: Routledge, 2001. 258–274.

Spillers, Hortense J. "Mama's Baby, Papa's Maybe: An American Grammar Book." *diacritics* (1987): 65–81.

Stabiner, Karen. *To Dance with the Devil: The New War on Breast Cancer: Politics, Power, People.* New York: Delta, 1998.

Steingraber, Sandra. "Apology to Audre Lorde, Never Sent." *Post-Diagnosis.* Ithaca: Firebrand Books, 1995. 38–40.

———. "The Environmental Link to Breast Cancer." *Breast Cancer: Society Shapes an Epidemic.* Ed. Anne S. Kasper and Susan J. Ferguson. New York: St. Martin's Press, 2000. 271–299.

———. "'If I Live to Be 90 Still Wanting to Say Something': My Search for Rachel Carson." *Confronting Cancer, Constructing Change: New Perspectives on Women and Cancer.* Ed. Midge Stocker. Chicago: Third Side Press, 1993. 181–199.

———. "Lifestyles Don't Kill. Carcinogens in Air, Food, and Water Do: Imagining Political Responses to Cancer." *Cancer as a Women's Issue: Scratching the Surface.* Ed. Midge Stocker. Chicago: Third Side Press, 1991. 91–102.

———. *Living Downstream: An Ecologist Looks at Cancer and the Environment.* Reading: Addison-Wesley, 1997.

———. "We All Live Downwind." *1 in 3: Women with Cancer Confront an Epidemic.* Ed. Judy Brady. Pittsburgh: Cleis Press, 1991. 36–48.

Stocker, Midge, ed. *Confronting Cancer, Constructing Change: New Perspectives on Women and Cancer.* Chicago: Third Side Press, 1993.

Stowe, Harriet Beecher. *Uncle Tom's Cabin.* 1852. New York: Oxford University Press, 1988.

Torgerson, Douglas. *The Promise of Green Politics: Environmentalism and the Public Sphere.* Durham: Duke University Press, 1999.

Turnbull, Eleanor M. "Effect of Basic Preventive Health Practices and Mass Media on the Practice of Breast Self-Examination." *Nursing Research* 27 (1978): 98–102.

Twombly, Renee. "After Long Island Study, Advocates Look for a Stronger Voice." *Journal of the National Cancer Institute* 94 (2002): 1349.

Underwood, Sandra Milton. "Breast Cancer Early Detection and Control: Strategies for Community Outreach." *Contemporary Issues in Breast Cancer.* Ed. Karen Hassey Dow. Boston: Jones & Bartlett, 1996. 185–191.

United States. Cong. House. Committee on Aging. *Breast Cancer Detection: The Need for a Federal Response.* 99th Cong., 1st sess., Washington: GPO, 23 October 1985.

———. Committee on Government Operations. *Thirty Years after Silent Spring: Status of EPA's Review of Older Pesticides.* 102nd Cong., 2nd sess., Washington: GPO, 23 July 1992.

———. Committee on Interstate and Foreign Commerce. *Concern about the Over Use of X-Rays, the Potential Health Hazards Posed by X-Rays and the Existing Levels of X-Ray Exposures Which We Now Consider Safe.* 95th Cong., 2nd sess., Washington: GPO, 11–14 July 1978.

———. Senate. Committee on Commerce. *Pesticide Research and Controls.* 88th Cong., 1st sess. Washington: GPO, 6 June 1963.

———. Committee on Government Operations. *Interagency Coordination in Environmental Hazards (Pesticides).* 88th Cong., 1st sess., pt. 1. Washington: GPO, 4 June 1963.

———. Committee on Labor and Public Welfare. *Examination on the Treatment of Breast Cancer, What Treatment Is Best, Where Physicians Differ, and the Risks and Costs Involved.* 94th Cong., 2nd sess. Washington: GPO,, 4 May 1976.

van Emden, Helmut F., and David B. Peakall. *Beyond Silent Spring: Integrated Pest Management and Chemical Safety.* London: Chapman & Hall, 1996.

Vig, Norman J., and Michael E. Kraft, eds. *Environmental Policy: New Directions for the Twenty-First Century.* Washington: CQ Press, 2000.

Villarosa, Linda, ed. *Body and Soul: The Black Women's Guide to Physical Health and Emotional Well-Being.* New York: HarperPerennial, 1994.

Walker, Bailus, Larry W. Figgs, and Sheila Hoar Zahm. "Differences in Cancer Incidence, Mortality, and Survival between African Americans and Whites." *Environmental Health Perspectives* 103, supp. 8 (1995): 275–281.

Warner, Michael. "The Mass Public and the Mass Subject." *The Phantom Public Sphere.* Ed. Bruce Robbins. Minneapolis: University of Minnesota Press, 1993. 234–256.

White, Evelyn C., ed. *The Black Women's Health Book: Speaking for Ourselves.* Seattle: Seal Press, 1990.

Whorton, James. *Before Silent Spring: Pesticides and Public Health in Pre-DDT America.* Princeton: Princeton University Press, 1974.

Writing Group for the Women's Health Initiative Investigators. "Risks and Benefits of Estrogen Plus Progestin in Healthy Post Menopausal Women: Principal Results from the Women's Health Initiative Randomized Controlled Trial." *Journal of the American Medical Association* 288 (2002): 321–333.

Yalom, Marilyn. *A History of the Breast.* New York: Knopf, 1997.

Yeazell, Ruth Bernard. Introduction. *The Death and Letters of Alice James.* Ed. Ruth Bernard Yeazell. Boston: Exact Change Press, 1997.

Young, Iris Marion. "Breasted Experience." *Throwing Like a Girl and Other Essays in*

Feminist Philosophy and Social Theory. Bloomington: Indiana University Press, 1990. 189–209.

Yúdice, George. "*Testimonio* and Postmodernism." *The Real Thing: Testimonial Discourse and Latin America.* Ed. Georg M. Gugelberger. Durham: Duke University Press, 1996. 42–57.

Zones, Jane Sprague. "Profits from Pain: The Political Economy of Breast Cancer." *Breast Cancer: Society Shapes an Epidemic.* Ed. Anne S. Kasper and Susan J. Ferguson. New York: St. Martin's Press, 2000. 119–151.

INDEX

Abramson Cancer Center, 148
Adams, Abigail, 2
Adams, John, 2
African Americans, xii, 17, 25, 71, 72, 102, 110, 114, 116, 117, 120, 125; activists, 126; autobiography and, 111, 112, 116–117; cancer incidence and mortality, 21, 82, 84, 124, 133, 143, 154; controlling body, 112, 113, 117, 119, 129, 139; controlling environment, 113, 137; health and well-being, 141; invisibility, 119–120; labor and, 137–138; lynchings of, 130; medical objectification of, 4; and myths about race and cancer, 63, 81–82; police violence and, 130, 132; stereotypes of, 20; survival of, 115, 123, 135; and women's bodies, 121, 130–131, 139, 141
Afrikaners, 114, 126
African National Congress, 128
Alexander, Elizabeth, 115, 131
Alexander, Shana, 80
American Cancer Society, 10, 16, 20, 63, 71, 82, 83, 84, 85, 89, 105, 117, 124, 142, 148. *See also* American Society for the Control of Cancer
American College of Radiology, 83
American College of Surgeons, 10
American Indians, 21
American Medical Association, 10, 19, 40–41, 49

American Society for the Control of Cancer, 16–17; Women's Field Army, 16–19. *See also* American Cancer Society
Anglin, Mary, 104
Arab/Israeli War of 1973, 89
Ashkenazi Jews, 23, 92, 109, 150
Asian/Pacific Islanders, 21; and myths about race and cancer, 63
Associated Women of the American Farm Bureau Federation, 17
atomic bomb, 33, 34, 35. *See also* Bikini atoll; Hiroshima; Nagasaki
atomic energy, 32–33, 37
Atomic Energy Commission, 54
atomic fallout, 30, 43, 53, 54; effects on fish and wildlife, 35; food chain and, 35
Audre Lorde Action Brigade, 142
Austin, Mary, 4
autobiography, 63, 65–66, 72, 76, 110, 111, 114, 137; bearing witness, 29, 73, 76, 84, 88, 112, 115, 126; diaries, xiii–xiv, 5, 113, 122–123, 126, 128, 131, 135–136; illness narratives, 73, 90; Internet, 5, 148–149; journals, 117, 122; magazines, 5, 11, 19, 20, 149; memoirs, 91–92, 96, 116; slave narratives, 112, 115, 116–117, 129; television, 5, 19; *testimonio*, 127–128, 132; testimony, 2, 73, 76, 77, 81, 94, 98, 104, 139, 152
Avery, Byllye, 141

About the Author

Marcy Jane Knopf-Newman is an assistant professor of English at Boise State University. She is the editor of *The Sleeper Wakes: Harlem Renaissance Stories by Women* and Jessie Fauset's *The Chinaberry Tree & Selected Writings*.